THE NEW
Sensual
MASSAGE

THE NEW Sensual MASSAGE

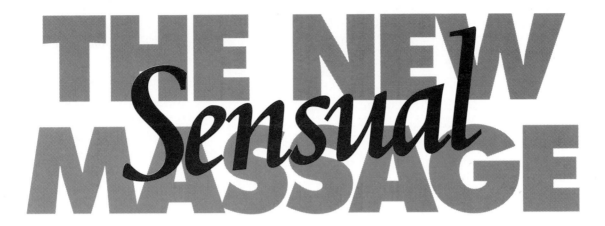

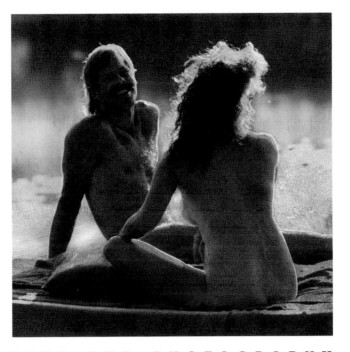

TEXT AND PHOTOGRAPHY
GORDON INKELES

BANTAM BOOKS
New York ♦ Toronto ♦ London ♦ Sydney ♦ Auckland

Library of Congress Cataloging-in-Publication Data
Inkeles, Gordon.
The new sensual massage/Gordon Inkeles.
    p.   cm.
ISBN 0-553-37092-8 (pbk.)
I. Massage.   I. Title.
RA780.5.I55 1992
615.8'22 — dc20   92-20126   CIP

Published simultaneously in the United States and Canada.

Acknowledgments

The New Sensual Massage was photographed
in the spring and summer of 1991, exactly
twenty years after *The Art of Sensual Massage*
photography sessions.

Jon Goodchild returned to design this new
book — it couldn't have been otherwise. Becky
Cabaza provided invaluable editorial guidance
at every turn. Karla Kaizoji Austin's illustrations show the interior of the body as a masseur sees it.

Special thanks to all those who helped
demonstrate the massage sequences: Brigette
Bartholomy, Susan Barton, Andy Camarda,
Kathy Compagno, Brian Harper, Little, Charlie
Mott, Robert Stepp, and Brigette Terry.

I am grateful to the people of Humboldt
County, California, who helped make this book
possible: Steve Dazey, Linda and Lieb Ostrow,
and Mark and Barbara Phelps generously
made their properties available for photography.
Scott Harrison did the photo processing and
pre-production work. Iris Schencke massaged
the manuscript for many hours and designed
the sets. Also, a heartfelt thank you to
Margaret Brown, Douglas Ingold, Linda
Loewenthal, Elaine Markson, Damian Sharp,
Katherine Sweet, and Lee Wakefield.

The New Sensual Massage was composed and
produced in Quark XPress by Robin Benjamin
at TBD Typography, San Rafael, CA.

Photographs included in Chapter 13 are
reprinted with permission from *Massage Magazine; Healing Arts Home Video,* Steve Adams and
Robert Foothorap; Body Support Systems, Inc.,
and Robert Jaffee; TouchAmerica and Robin
Zill; Don Payne and Living Earth Crafts.

*Bantam Books are published by Bantam Books,
a division of Bantam Doubleday Dell Publishing
Group, Inc. Its trademark, consisting of the words
"Bantam Books" and the portrayal of a rooster, is
Registered in U.S. Patent and Trademark Office and
in other countries. Marca Registrada. Bantam Books,
1540 Broadway, New York, New York 10036.*

For my son
Matthew Damian Inkeles

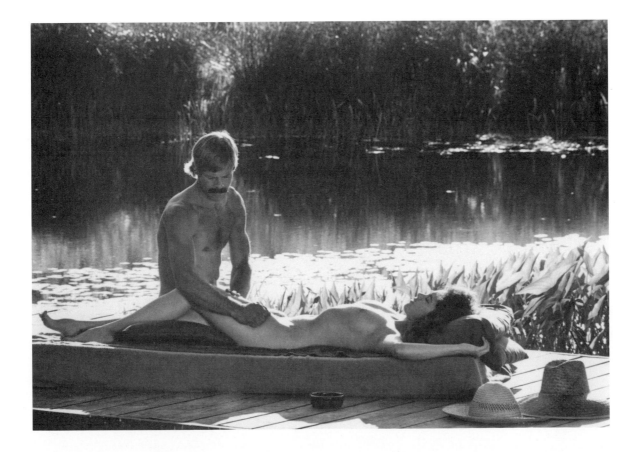

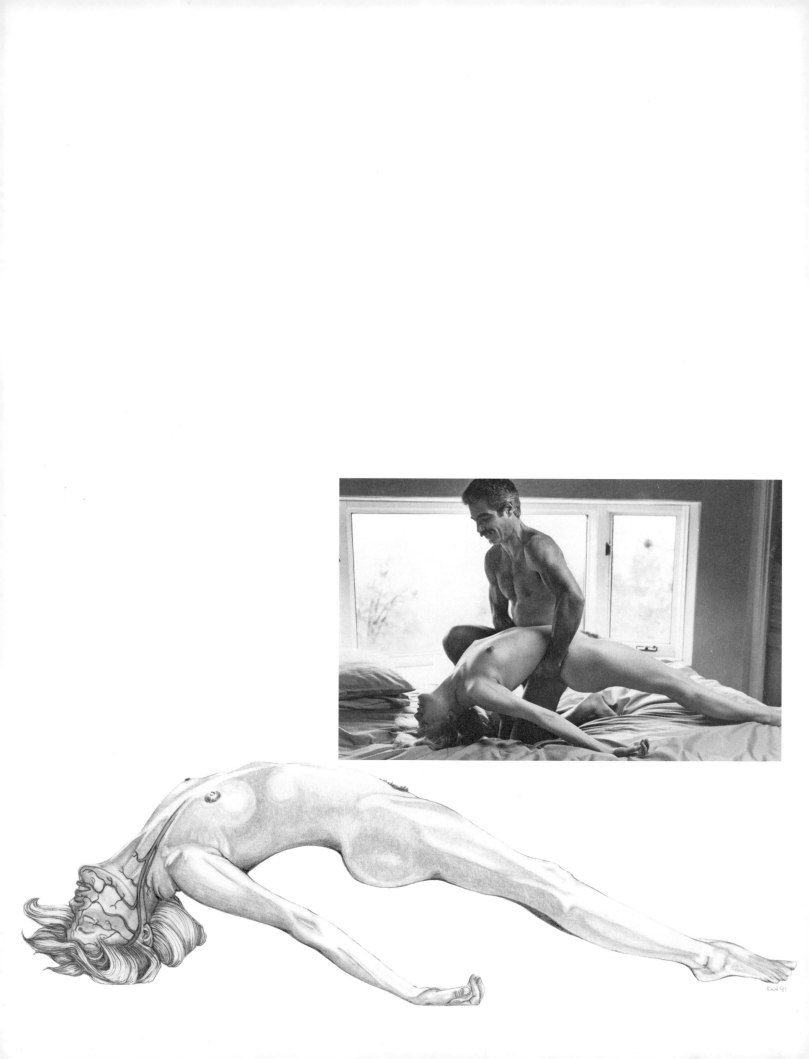

Contents

Twenty Years of Sensual Massage

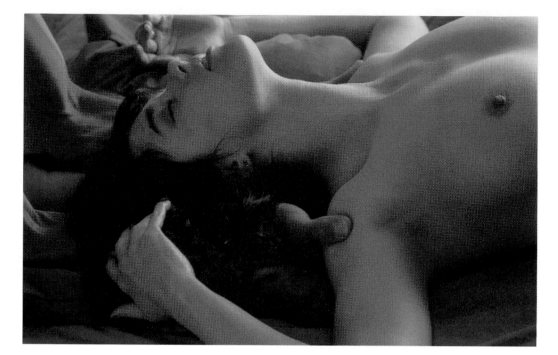

I wrote *The Art of Sensual Massage* twenty years ago to demystify massage and liberate it from the cold, impersonal clinical model. The practice of massage, in those days, had been handed over to a small group of self-appointed scientific experts who took pains to make it as complicated and unfriendly as possible. If you were brave enough to try massage (usually after a muscle-wrenching accident), you reclined on what looked suspiciously like an operating table. Shelves of ominous devices

— trusses, syringes, bandages, and medications — filled the room. The intercom blared, someone was hemorrhaging in Ward Three. A big nurse in her starched white uniform loomed over you, overworked and scowling. You had made a mess of yourself; now she was expected to fix it. Adjusting the overhead fluorescent fixture to eliminate all shadows, she reached for a bottle of ice-cold alcohol. You twisted your head to the side, gritting your teeth, as her rough hands took hold of your imperfect body. . . .

So in 1972 the score was Puritans 10, Humans 0 . . . but another kind of massage waited in the wings. Practiced everywhere on earth since biblical times, its adherents held no clinical degrees and didn't depend on Latin and German to describe their techniques. Yes, the skull had temporal and parietal lobes, but it also had natural handles at the back of the neck and the chin that allowed you to turn the head in a single smooth uninterrupted motion. Hands and feet had their own handles, so did the arms and legs. Fingertips fit perfectly between the eyes and eyebrows, thumbs filled the spaces between the vertebrae, and the curvature of the pelvic bone perfectly accommodated the heel of the hand. People fit together in unexpected ways almost as though the human body had been designed to be massaged.

I got my first massage nearly thirty years ago in a candle-lit San Francisco Victorian. I can remember it as though it were yesterday. On a pale gray summer evening while the mournful cry of distant foghorns drifted in from San Francisco Bay, a woman I hardly knew spent two hours spreading pleasure over every inch of my body. Afterward, I felt distinct physical pleasure in places I hadn't thought capable of feeling much at all. My feet, liberated from the tyranny of leather shoes, were suddenly warm and alive. The muscles of my face surrendered their hidden tensions — I actually looked different. All that night and throughout the following

day, a warm, friendly feeling seemed to envelop my body. Every muscle and joint worked more smoothly. Without sex, without actually doing a single thing, I had experienced two hours of uninterrupted physical pleasure. I simply hadn't realized anything like that was on the menu in life.

A first sensual massage transforms virtually every part of your body. For a while, you walk around simply feeling good from head to toe, glowing. And then you want to learn how to give the experience to others.

I wrote this book to give the reader an hour of the most gratifying physical pleasure. If *The Art of Sensual Massage* was an appetizer, an introduction to the pleasures of sensual massage, this new book is meant to be a banquet, a sensual feast. For twenty years, I've been thinking about the full-body massage that follows. From hundreds of possibilities on every part of the body, I've selected the popular strokes that everyone loves.

What most people want out of life, regardless of age, background, education, appearance, or cultural bias is to have a good time. An hour of *The New Sensual Massage* is guaranteed to get almost anyone there.

GORDON INKELES
Miranda, California

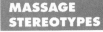

♦ Massage has outgrown two stereotypes in the last twenty years, the sado-masochistic and the sexual. Bowing to puritanical pressures, practitioners once viewed the body as an evil place that had to be tortured back into good health. Massage was a painful ordeal. You deserved to suffer and your massage therapist never let you forget it. The notion

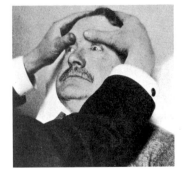

that pleasure itself could be therapeutic was dismissed as frivolous, even sinful.

The massage parlor is going the way of the dance hall as a clumsy front for prostitution. When everybody learned how to dance, a new code word had to be chosen. Real massage, now offered in resorts, hotels, and small towns from coast-to-coast, has found a place at the center of American life.

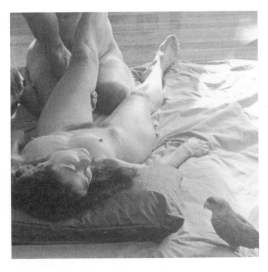

PART I

Start Massaging Tonight

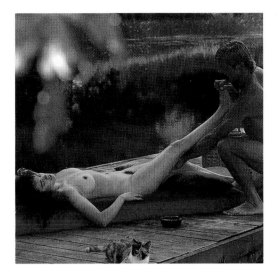

CHAPTER I

Atmosphere, Preparation, Oils

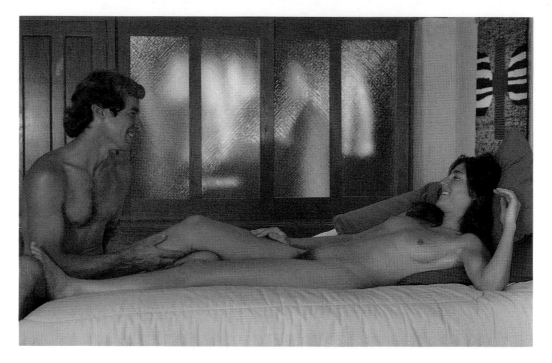

Ten minutes from now, without opening an anatomy book or enrolling in a class, you can begin to give your partner one of life's most delicious experiences: a full-body massage. You won't need to practice strange exercises or develop unused muscles. Think of massage as educated touching. You were born to do massage, to give pleasure with your hands.

Massage works the first time you try it. Even though your technique may not be perfect, remember that people love being touched. Simply making unhurried contact with your partner's body initiates a warm, deeply relaxing feeling. This book is about turning that feeling into happiness.

As you begin, watch for the special smile that signals the profound release of tension masseurs know so well. Listen carefully and you may hear your partner's blissful moans. During massage the world seems to slow down to its natural pace; peace becomes a tangible sensation.

Many specific health benefits are indicated throughout the book but don't wait for a bad back or aching shoulders to try massage. Everything you do will spread pleasure; no further justification is needed.

Massage says: You are *here*, whole, and alive.

Choose a warm (at least seventy degrees Fahrenheit on the massage *surface*), quiet place to do massage. If you decide to warm a section of a room, use a quiet electric heater. Noisy fans that cycle on and off will distract both of you. Your partner will get the most out of her massage on a moderately firm, padded surface. A few inches of foam rubber, even a sleeping bag, will support her body nicely while you press down. A deep spongy mattress yields too much and makes it awkward for you to move around. Avoid billowy surfaces like water beds and giant pillows, which turn back massage into a rolling, pitching affair. Cover your massage surface and small pillows with a soft, friendly material like cotton or silk. Since your partner will experience massage with her eyes closed, texture matters much more than color.

Give yourself room to move around your partner without knocking over essential tools like towels and oil.

Your hands will be in continuous contact with your partner's body from the moment you begin massage to the end of the last stroke. Trim and file your fingernails and wash your hands in very hot water before you begin massage. The heat will soften any calluses and make your hands feel smooth and inviting.

Your hands must be warm before you make contact with your partner. If the hot water doesn't do it, press both hands into your armpits, fingers outstretched, and fold your arms down against them. You will then feel something close to what your partner feels when you touch him. Your body heat will warm your hands in a minute or two.

TEMPERATURE

◆ Eliminate drafts. While you do massage, your partner does nothing at all. She will be far more temperature-sensitive than you. No matter what strokes you use, any chill will immediately cause the muscles to tighten. Massaging in a cold room is like trying to cook on a pilot light; your partner must be warm for massage to succeed.

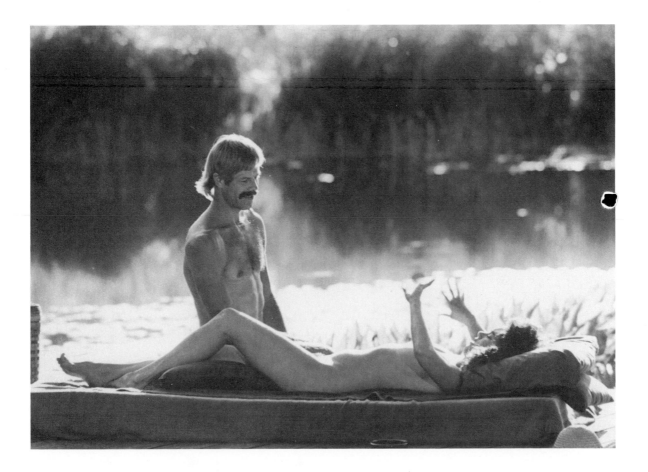

Setting the Mood

Massage creates an exquisite range of sensations that cannot be duplicated anywhere else in life. As the body surrenders its defenses and opens up to the world around it, your partner will begin to experience long-forgotten nuances of feeling. You should regard anything that will interrupt the mood — and shatter a massage — as a violation. Unplug the phone and lock the door. Make sure children and pets are looked after. Before you begin, spend a few moments sitting quietly in your massage area simply looking around and listening. Do what you can to eliminate bright lights and noise.

Controlling Sound

Since your partner experiences massage with her eyes closed, her sense of hearing will be particularly acute.

In a perfectly quiet room she will hear the primal skin-on-skin sounds of massage. But unless your massage area is truly silent, appliance noise, street sounds, and through-the-wall vibrations will intrude. Rain provides a great screen of sonic peace, a perfect background for massage. And, of course, so does the right music.

Choose something soothing that will complement, not compete with, the mood. Find out what your partner likes and set up an audio source (tape, compact disc, or noncommercial radio) that will play *without interruption* right through the massage. To be certain the music won't stop suddenly, you may want to use a VCR as an audio tape recorder. Simply substituting an audio source for the television provides an inexpensive way to record your own long-playing music for massage program. Whether the tape is played back over a stereo or television, you get at least two hours of continuous music with surprisingly good sound quality. Generally, background music for massage works best at lower volume levels.

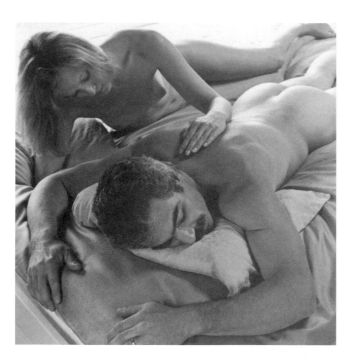

Arranging the Tools

Think about three tools — oil, pillows, and towels. Put them where they can be reached easily throughout the massage. Everyone loves a generous fluffy towel that feels as luxurious and warm as it looks. Small towels work over small parts of the body like the hands and feet but tend to scrub at your partner on the back or chest. Keep a couple of larger towels on hand. Even the most sure-footed masseur can knock over a bowl of massage oil. A plastic squeeze bottle, while less attractive, protects you and your partner from messy oil spills.

Manners

Be warm. Your initial approach begins to establish the mood. Since everything you do is transmitted directly to your partner's body, there are no wasted strokes in a good massage. Forget about time limits, clocks, or schedules. Massage should have no frustrating moments. Avoid a brusque, super-efficient manner. Speak softly. Move slowly. Keep your hands warm.

"At Ohio University School, one researcher conducted an experiment in which he fed rabbits high-cholesterol diets and methodically petted a special group of them; the petted rabbits had a 50 percent lower rate of arteriosclerosis than similarly fed but unpetted rabbits. . . .

"(The librarian) brushes a student's hand lightly as she returns a library card. Then the student is followed outside and asked to fill out a questionnaire about the library that day. Among other questions, the student is asked if the librarian smiled, and if she touched him. In fact, the librarian had not smiled, but the student reports that she did, although he says she did not touch him. . . . soon a pattern becomes clear: those students who have been subconsciously touched report much more satisfaction with the library and life in general."

Diane Ackerman, *A Natural History of the Senses* (New York: Random House, 1990), pp. 121, 122–23.

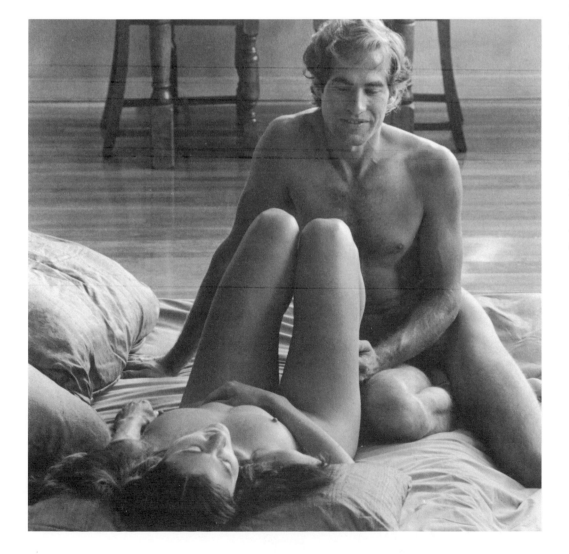

◆ Never do anything that causes pain. If it hurts, stop. If it keeps hurting, don't continue with massage until your partner sees a doctor.

Don't massage if your partner has an infection or fever, skin eruptions or bruises, inflamed joints, sensitive veins, a tumor, lump, or cyst.

Generosity

If you must think during massage, think about how you can be generous — there are so many opportunities. Generally, the more you do a stroke, the better it feels. Repeat the long circulation strokes (see page 18) at least ten times, other strokes three times.

Listen to your partner's requests; watch for the moans of pleasure, the secret smiles. Remember, a few extra minutes of friction (see page 20) on stiff shoulder muscles may be appreciated for days to come.

Massage has a simple program: Give your partner what she wants.

Rhythm and Touch

Big strokes and little strokes move at the same speed. A steady rhythm establishes the mood as surely as the individual strokes. Massage is hypnosis of the body.

Do not break body contact. From the first back stroke to the end of the massage, remaining in continuous physical contact with your partner matters more than fine points of technique. Make contact during breaks and when moving from one part of the body to another. If you need both hands elsewhere for a moment, use your knee, foot, or even the side of an arm, to stay in touch. After a while, your partner's tactile awareness, her sensate focus, simply follows your hands. Your touch becomes a physical bond between the two of you. Don't break it.

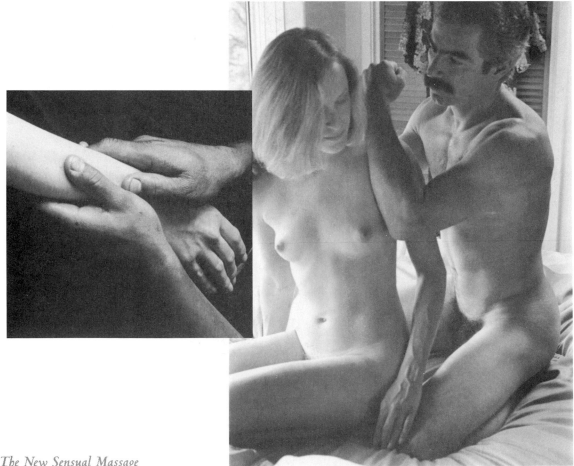

Oiling

Oiling makes every massage movement (except friction and percussion) easier. You will oil every part of the body except the scalp. Most light vegetable oils like safflower and sesame seed work as well as the high-priced "commercial" products. At room temperatures when it liquifies, coconut oil is ideal for massage. Olive and peanut oil are too thick.

Massage oil feels best if it's warmer than your partner's body temperature. Before you begin, immerse a bottle of oil in a pot of warm water to bring it up to a comfortable temperature. Keeping your oil in a small plastic squeeze bottle will prevent spills.

Oiling puts you in contact with your partner's body, thus signaling the beginning of massage. Always think of it as part of the massage, not a separate act.

Add oil to your own hands — never pour it directly onto your partner's body.

To maintain contact, press the back of your fingers against your partner's body while you pour oil into your palm. Spread the oil in broad flat-hand strokes to cover the whole area you plan to massage. Oil allows your hands to move smoothly without pulling at the skin. Too much oil and your hands will skid all over the body; too little and the massage degenerates into jerky scrubbing motions. Add just enough to feel your partner's skin as your hands glide over it. Whenever you feel the skin drying out during massage, add additional oil. If you need to reach for the bottle, maintain contact with your knee or the side of an arm.

Don't confuse massage oiling with applying suntan lotion, which is generally rubbed onto the body as impersonally as possible (lest one be accused of making a sexual advance). Remember, most people haven't been gently oiled by another human being since early childhood. Back then, oiling the body was an exquisitely tender ceremony. It still is.

SCENT

◆ Scent your oil with a few drops of lemon juice or your partner's favorite essence. If you burn incense in the room, choose a complementary scent and keep the smokier varieties away from your massage area. Take a moment to discuss your partner's preferences before you make a choice. The right scent goes directly to the brain, unmediated by thought, and sets a pleasant mood for hours to come. The wrong incense, however, can bring on an allergic reaction, which will spoil the massage. If you're not sure how to proceed, the universally popular lemon-scented oil may provide all the aroma you need.

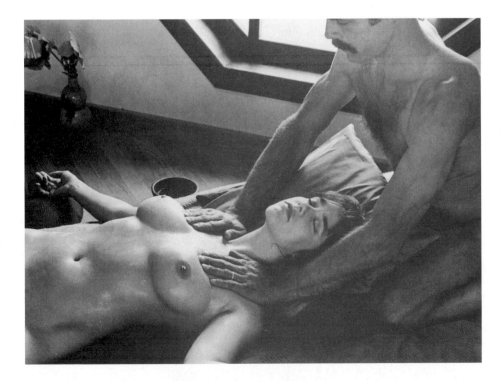

♦ Divide a full-body massage into two unequal parts: the front and back of the body. Relax the back first, for about twenty minutes, and the rest of the body will follow.

Contact between adults is rigidly controlled in our society — we insist on facing people who touch us. Most adults haven't experienced continuous physical contact on the back of the body for years, even decades. We may struggle against the joyless Puritan ethic but generally, we do it with the front of our bodies — we conceded the back in childhood. Fully half the body, from the back of the neck to the bottom of the foot, sleepwalks though life locked in a bizarre kind of tactile deprivation. Massaging the back of the body changes that, once and for all.

A Massage Map

Keep massage simple when you're learning. The pages that follow present dozens of different strokes but you don't have to learn them all to give a complete body massage — repetition of a few well-executed strokes counts more than variety for its own sake.

Each chapter begins with a circulation stroke that spreads sensation over the whole part of the body you're about to massage. Make sure to do that essential stroke, then add one of the more expansive kneading movements (see page 17), usually a full-hand variation, that travels easily. After at least three passes over the whole region, focus your kneading wherever you feel tightness and keep at it until you feel the muscles begin to relax — usually, a minute or two.

After kneading, choose from a variety of proven strokes in each chapter: friction (see page 20) to focus on aches and pains; compression (see page 26) to spread deep sensations; passive exercise (see page 24) to work the joints; and percussion (see page 22) to wake up an unfeeling body. On the limbs, chest, and back, end with one of the authoritative full-body circulation variations that moves sensation from one part of the body to another.

Finish the back with a full-body stroke starting on the ankles.

Finish the right leg by holding one hand on your partner's right calf while touching the left calf. Then move to the other side of your partner's body.

Finish the legs with a full-body stroke from the ankles to the shoulders.

1. back

2. back of the right leg
3. back of the left leg

4. back of the right foot
5. back of the left foot

Give the smaller body parts as much attention as the larger ones. Complete the hands and feet with a brushing movement (see pages 75 and 133) that will transfer sensation to the ends of the fingertips and toes.

If you begin and end a massage with strong circulation strokes and include several minutes of kneading and compression, you will have completed a basic fluid release sequence (see page 13). Your partner will feel the difference immediately . . . and for hours afterward.

If you need to rest or you're not sure how to proceed, move to a compression stroke that focuses sensation on a single spot. Don't break contact with your partner. When you're ready to move on, begin rotating your hands in small circles. Let compression blend with the next movement you plan to do.

During massage your partner develops an intensely personal awareness. Her attention, usually focused on the world outside her body, becomes purely sensual; she follows your hands wherever they go. Break contact, even for a moment, and she will feel abandoned.

Pick strokes from Part 2 to create your own full-body massage or simply do them all in the order they appear. If you choose a basic approach of four or five strokes on each part of the body, repeat each one twenty or thirty times. The more you vary the strokes, the less repetition you will need — generally, ten times for circulation strokes, three for most others. Including all the strokes in Part 2 will create an unforgettable full-body massage that lasts an hour or more.

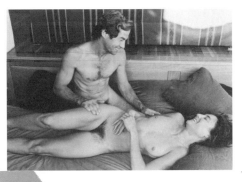

While holding the right shoulder, reach across and grasp the left shoulder. Then move to the opposite side of your partner's body.

Massage the head from above.

Your partner should turn over midway through the foot massage.

6. *front of the right foot*

7. *front of the left foot*

8. *front of the right leg*

9. *front of the left leg*

10. *chest*

11. *right arm*

12. *right hand*

13. *left arm*

14. *left hand*

15. *head*

CHAPTER 2

Inside the Body

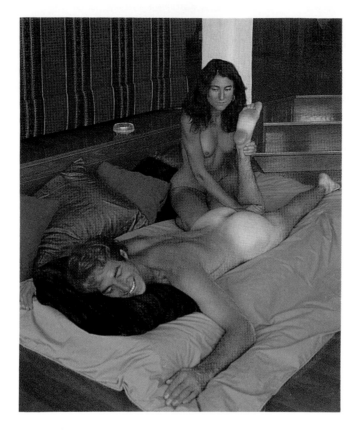

At the end of a complete massage, virtually every part of the body feels restored and energized. The natural high that lasts for hours isn't your partner's imagination; inside the body great changes have taken place. The effects begin on the surface of the skin.

That massaged babies grow faster, are more even-tempered, and generally prosper is now universally recognized. Your partner will testify to the profound changes that adults experience during massage. One hour of peace stabilizes the mind as well as the body. A steady emotional calm, similar to the state people achieve after deep meditation, takes hold, banishing nervous tension. You begin to think more clearly. A well-massaged body becomes more alert and responsive.

Throughout the book, Karla Kaizoji Austin's illustrations furnish a masseur's-eye view inside the body. Specific tissues that actually feel the effect of each stroke are separated from the mass of anatomical background detail. You will see how to relieve pressure on the nerves that supply the hands by relaxing congested areas at the wrist and shoulder. Here are the blood vessels that contract during headaches, the muscles of the abdomen that begin on the back, the exquisitely sensitive nerve paths on the inside of the legs, and the ligaments that stretch when you flex a joint. Each illustration matches a specific photograph, providing an anatomical map of your partner's body in the precise position that you massage it.

Circulation

Massage helps two fluids pass through the body: blood and lymph. Simple circulation movements will triple the flow rate of both substances, while toning the vascular system. Your hands help do the heart's work by pressing open capillary valves in the limbs. Post-massage blood pressure reductions of 10% or more have been measured. Focusing for five minutes on a single part of the body, like your partner's aching neck, boosts the blood supply by up to 85%. This in turn increases the oxygen content of the tissues by 10 to 15%, which acts as a natural analgesic or pain control.

The effects on the lymph system are even more dramatic. Acidic wastes and toxins that might take many days to leave the body are dispersed in minutes. More on that in a moment.

Skin

Dead brittle skin is swept aside allowing the living tissue below to breathe freely. You can feel the difference the moment massage begins. Rough skin becomes more supple. As subcutaneous circulation is stimulated, the skin, even the hair (via scalp massage, page 141), acquires a healthy glow.

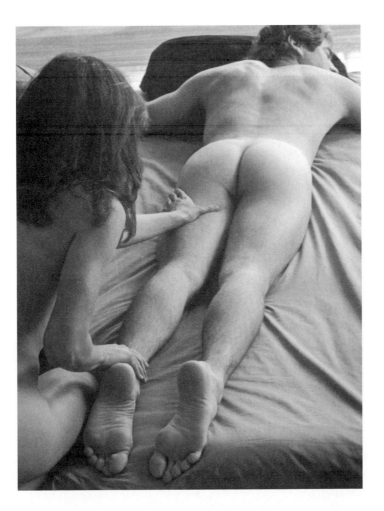

THE OLDEST THERAPY

◆ Massage is drugless therapy, perhaps the oldest therapy, predating most medicines, spirits, and stimulants. In the earliest medical records it is "prescribed" by Hippocrates, Galen, the Sanskrit Ayur-Veda, by healers in Egypt, China, Peru, Siberia, the American Southwest, and the Pacific Islands for a wide range of problems we now try to solve by popping a pill . . . or two. In fact, massage was practiced widely by physicians until the turn of the century when it became more cost-effective to write a prescription than to lay your hands on a patient.

In the nineteenth century, Americans who could manage to be massaged usually were. "Indeed, during my [massage] practice in Washington," said Dr. Hartvig Nissen of the Harvard Medical School, "I frequently had to shut off the light in the White House, telling the officers at the door, as I left, that the President was asleep." A hundred years earlier a lengthy team massage by twelve Hawaiian women permanently banished the famous Captain Cook's chronic sciatica. These old-timers surely had as much pressure to deal with as any modern worker, but they chose massage instead of drugs.

Muscles

Facial wrinkles are caused by poor muscle tone in subcutaneous tissues, not by a defect in the skin itself. This is why facial creams, no matter how rarefied and expensive, fail while simple fingertip massage techniques can work wonders. The fluid release effect creates an even more dramatic change: the astonishing difference in the recovery rate of large muscles before and after massage.

Nerves and Brain

Massage reaches the nervous system first. Soothe the nerves, and the rest of the body will follow. Light to mild pressures stimulate the nerves, while heavy pressures will sedate them. Generally, women's nerves are more sensitive than men's and will require less pressure. Acidic wastes irritate the nerves, causing everything from moodiness to muscle cramps. Clear the system with fluid release strokes, techniques that squeeze acidic wastes out of the tissues, and the nerves are the first to benefit.

Although the brain itself feels nothing — merely registering feelings that originate elsewhere — it works much better on fresh oxygen. By oxygenating the brain, you can transform your partner's mood.

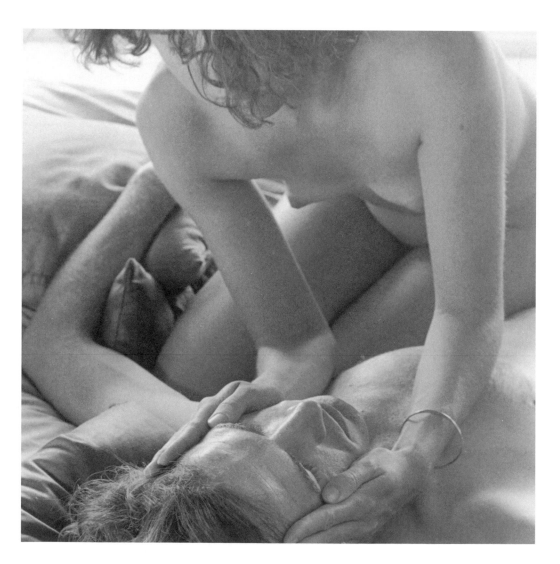

The Fluid Release Effect

When the exhaust gases, toxins, and wastes produced by metabolism remain within the body, stress is generated. Since it is impossible to escape from fatigue, anxiety, or depression if the muscles are bathed in toxins and acids, masseurs see stress primarily as a chemical, not a psychological, problem. You can't talk your way out of it and pills only mask the effects. You have to go directly to the body to get rid of stress. Happily, certain massage sequences will virtually eliminate tension-causing chemicals. These strokes bring about the amazing fluid release effect — wherein massage actually helps the body rid itself of the fluids that keep muscles perpetually tense.

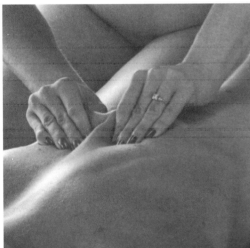

Simple massage routines you can learn in minutes will dramatically accelerate the body's natural cleansing process. The lymph system, which might normally take days, even weeks, to refresh itself, is squeezed out like a sponge — in minutes. Urinalysis reveals that nitrogen, sugar, inorganic phosphorus, and sodium chloride, the very substances that cause fatigue, are expelled from the body at accelerated rates up to one full week after a single massage session. But getting rid of nasty acidic gunk is only one part of the fluid release effect. As wastes and lactic acid, the by-product of exercise, are cleared from the tissues, oxygen-rich blood floods into the muscles. Suddenly, nagging aches and pains disappear, fatigue vanishes, and a sense of well-being takes its place. Massage as drugless therapy.

Continue fluid release massage on a specific set of muscles for fifteen minutes and you will begin to understand why so many Olympic teams refuse to leave home without their masseurs. After the massage, muscle recovery rates actually double and work output increases by more than 100%.

Use fluid release strokes to neutralize the chemical source of stress and reverse the vasoconstriction effect. Massage breaks the vicious cycle of tension.

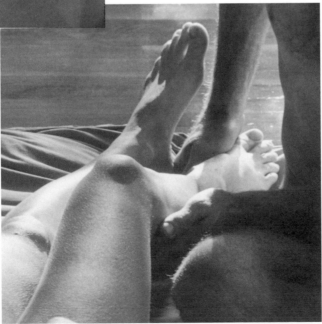

CONTROLLING STRESS

♦ Masseurs seek to reduce stress by working on the body, rather than the mind. Rarely can you talk anyone out of their tension. During stress (the "fight" impulse in animals), the vasoconstriction effect causes the muscles to tighten all over the body while the vascular system slows down. The blood supply to surface tissues is drastically reduced, resulting in the familiar pallid complexion that haunts perpetually stressed individuals. Vasoconstriction also slows the metabolism of acidic wastes. Chemical irritants remain trapped in the muscles for hours, even days — thus causing more stress. Animals, of course, expect to fight and get it over with. Over-stressed people tend to stay that way until something snaps, often landing themselves in a hospital emergency room.

Stress generated in specific parts of the body — such as aching feet, a stiff neck, or a pounding head — can be controlled by focusing three- and four-minute sequences on the tensed muscles that are causing the problem. As stiffened muscles give up their tension, you will hear your partner's breathing relax.

Fluid release sequences remove acidic wastes, breaking the cycle of stress, and the body returns to its natural peaceful state. This is one of the things human hands can do: ease pain.

Master Strokes

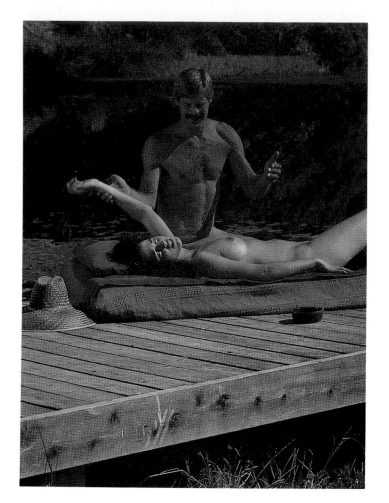

A little feedback at the beginning of a massage will focus your technique on your partner's personal needs. After a while, however, even a short conversation becomes distracting; words come between your partner and the feeling. Soon after you begin stroking, she will close her eyes and fall silent. A few minutes into the massage you may be wondering where to go next but afraid to ask.

Generally, what people want at any moment during a massage is more of the same. If it's a first massage, most of your partner's body may not have been touched by another human being for years; each new stroke is like presenting a starving man with a feast. If massage has a program, a master plan, it is simply this: *Be generous, let the feeling go on.*

When your partner's thoughts center on the hundreds of sensations that make up a full-body massage, she begins to feel things in unexpected ways. Gradually, as her body becomes an instrument of purely sensual pleasure, your massage becomes the full focus of her attention — she simply follows your hands. Everything you do is noticed, every sensation registers. At that point you no longer *do* massage, you *conduct* it; her body, fine-tuned like a great symphony orchestra, responds to every nuance of feeling created by your hands. This is the point of the six Master Strokes, to show you how to create that delicious mood and prolong it for an hour or more.

The Master Strokes are circulation, kneading, friction, compression, passive exercise, and percussion.

Strokes never begin and end abruptly; they flow into each other so what your partner feels is a single wave of sensation moving across the body. On the back of the knee, for example, you can create a seamless transfer of sensation between two very different Master Strokes. During leg flexing, a passive exercise (see page 24), your hand at the back of the knee serves as an anchor, a kind of "stop" to prevent your partner's leg from being flexed too far. The hand that actually flexes the leg creates the sensation. However, once your partner's leg is lowered to the massage surface for the final time a curious transfer of sensation occurs. Suddenly he becomes aware of a gentle pressure on the back of the knee. Make no mistake about it, having the back of the knee cupped gently but firmly is a unique experience for most adults — breaking the contact abruptly will create a tangible sense of abandonment.

(see page 24)

DO

♦ Put towels and oil where you can reach them easily
♦ Grant your partner's requests
♦ Maintain physical contact throughout the massage
♦ Ask for feedback on stroke and pressure preferences
♦ Appear confident and organized
♦ Vanish quietly when the massage is over

DON'T

♦ Massage while your partner does something else
♦ Comment on how tense your partner seems to be
♦ Break contact or abandon the massage if you are interrupted
♦ Randomly explore a body — people dislike being probed
♦ Start conversations, especially about somebody's problems

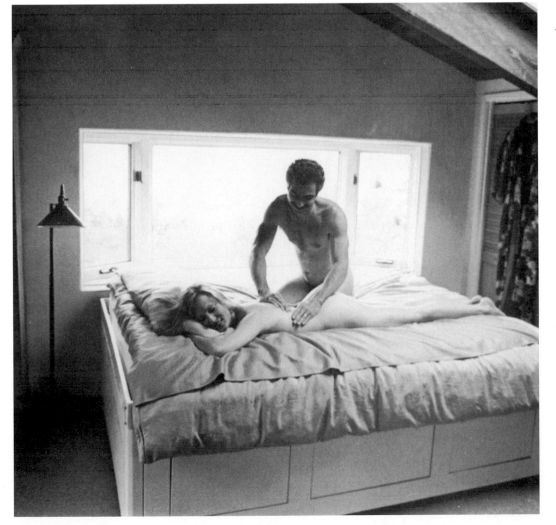

Transitions become opportunities to be generous, to extend a sensual moment rather than break it off. Continuing on the back of the knee, press down on your contact hand with the hand that was holding the ankle and begin compression, a simple hand-over-hand circling movement that either moves down the leg to the bottom of the foot or up onto the muscled thigh and buttocks. (As you move up onto thicker muscles, increase the pressure but be sure to end the stroke well below the bottom of the rib cage where a portion of the kidney is exposed.) You've now moved smoothly from one stroke, eg: flexing, into another, compression.

Your goal is always the same: to grant your partner an hour or more of uninterrupted physical pleasure. The Master Strokes provide you with simple techniques to extend the pleasure anywhere on your partner's body.

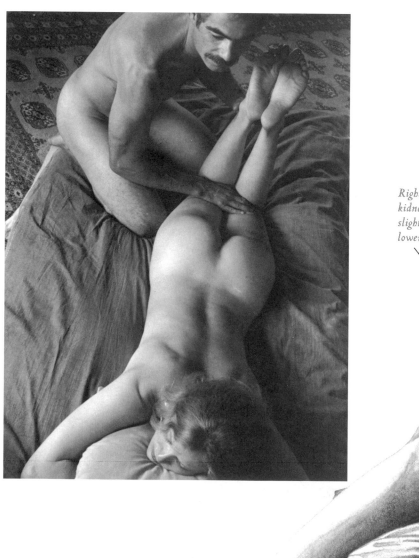

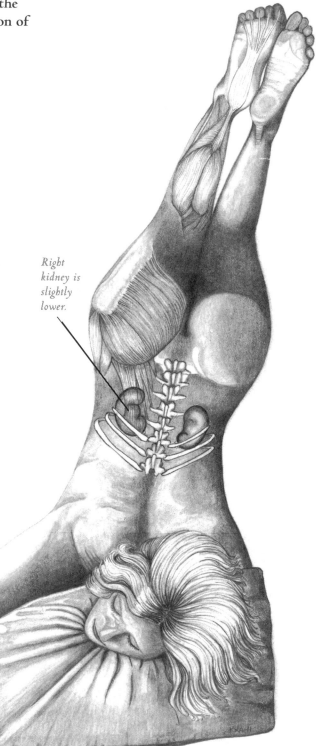

Right kidney is slightly lower.

Kneading

Kneading is the centerpiece of your full-body massage. From the scalp to the toes you will return to this essential stroke again and again. People simply can't get enough of being kneaded. On large fleshy areas like the thigh, knead with the full surface of your hand. Elsewhere where tissues are thinner, use your fingertips or thumbs. Lift a fold of flesh and squeeze gently as you knead.

Learn kneading one hand at a time. Make ten rhythmic circles with your right hand (left, if you're left-handed), picking up a fold of flesh with your thumb and letting it go each time you complete the circle. Then make ten identical circles with your other hand, concentrating on the same spot. Now circle over the same spot with both hands, picking up a fold of flesh with the left thumb whenever the right thumb is open and vice versa. The thumb is the key to superbly satisfying kneading. Open and close it as you pick up and release the squeezed flesh. When you knead smaller areas like the hands and feet, the thumbs become even more important. Grasp your partner's hand with four fingers and circle with your thumbs pressing down as you turn.

Avoid jerky, back-and-forth motions. Whether you move across the body or focus on a single spot, knead in smooth rhythmic circles. It becomes effortless after a while, a kind of tactile music. Feel the interior muscles roll off your fingertips. Your partner feels a delightful penetrating sensation that literally rolls across the body.

- Stay with a comfortable rhythm
- Keep your fingers together
- Use your thumbs to pick up flesh
- Move in tight circles
- Knead the same spot with both hands

DON'T

- Rush
- Pinch
- Jerk
- Poke
- Hesitate

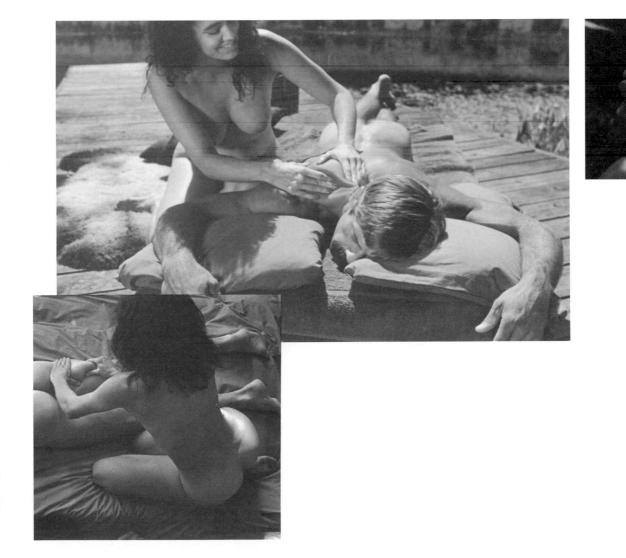

Circulation

Circulation strokes, the first ones performed in many massage sequences, travel up and down a limb and from one end of the chest or back to the other. Full-body circulation movements extend from the toes to the shoulders, spreading deep sensation everywhere.

This luxurious sequence leaves your partner with a feeling of suppleness and lightness that will radiate to the extremities of her body. It's the perfect intro-

duction to any massage. Normally, in a full-body massage, you will repeat a circulation sequence ten times. Repeat it three times if you want to make a truly smashing first impression.

Make contact from the tips of your fingers to the base of your palms. Push forward, molding your hands to the changing shape of your partner's body. Pull back at the top end of the stroke, making superficial contact with your fin-

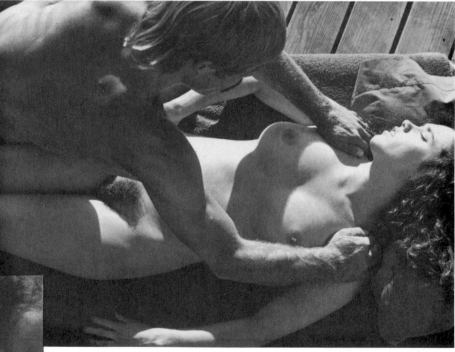

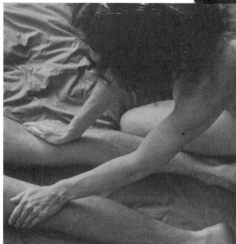

gertips. Press down while moving toward the heart and tiny capillary valves will open and close under your hands. The valves open in only one direction — toward the heart. Each time you press up the arms or legs, sticky valves are forced open. Oxygen-rich blood floods into every part of the body between your hands and your partner's heart, producing the light, exhilarating feeling everyone gets during massage. Circulation strokes improve your partner's mood.

In massage, stress is treated as a chemical imbalance rather than a purely mental one. If your cells are bathed in nasty acidic gunk, neither pills nor exercise will help you relax. The extraordinary fluid release effect (see page 13), which eliminates tension-causing chemicals that collect in the body's tissues, begins and ends with a massive circulation sequence. Circulation stimulates the venous and lymphatic systems simultaneously, increasing blood and lymph flow without speeding up the heart, an effect that cannot be achieved outside of massage.

◆ During circulation, keep your hands relaxed and supple so your fingers and palm can mold themselves to the changing shape of your partner's body. This is a luxurious movement—be generous. Let your circulation strokes spill out a bit, up onto the shoulder tops from the arms and down to the feet when massaging your partner's legs. Be ready to add extra oil on hairy parts of the body and dry skin. Circulation strokes should flow smoothly without pulling at the skin.

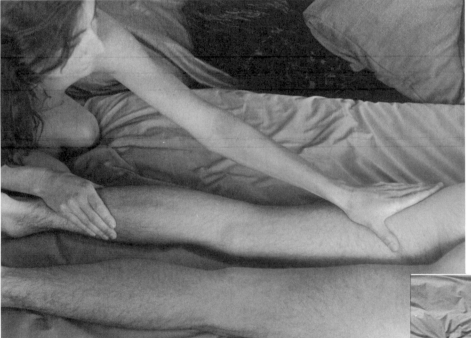

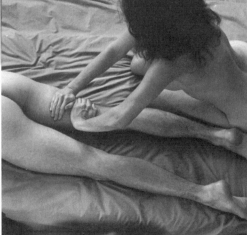

◆ Surface Friction: Keep your fingers apart, hands bent at the wrists. Brush the fingers back and forth. Use light pressure to warm the surface of the skin.

◆ Muscle Friction: Keep your fingers together, circle with your fingertips on visible muscles. If necessary, use an anchor hand to stabilize the body. Follow the contour of large muscle groups.

◆ Deep Friction: Use this intense version of muscle friction to reach into the body's largest joints at the hips and shoulders. Anchor every stroke before you begin. Don't rush the stroke; fatigue will slow you down quickly.

Friction

If your partner is nervous about trying massage, start with a short friction sequence. These easy-to-learn strokes provide deep direct pressure, a kind of instant massage that you can do with little preparation. Friction sends a fundamental message that is understood instinctively by all mammals: Rubbing the body produces relief. Since oil is unnecessary, friction works almost anywhere. In fact, a basic sequence will have some effect straight through clothing. "On-site" massage practitioners use friction on tense office workers right in the workplace.

But like every other massage stroke, friction works best if your hands meet naked skin and a recumbent body. The crude attempts at shoulder friction in the movies — invariably while a stressed character drives a car or makes a phone call — always seem, at best, like a polite gesture. As long as the head's great weight must be supported by the shoulders instead of, say, a pillow, massage will have little effect.

Think of massage as an antidote to the over-scheduled life. It shouldn't be rushed, abbreviated, or combined with other activities. Your partner doesn't "do" massage, he experiences it.

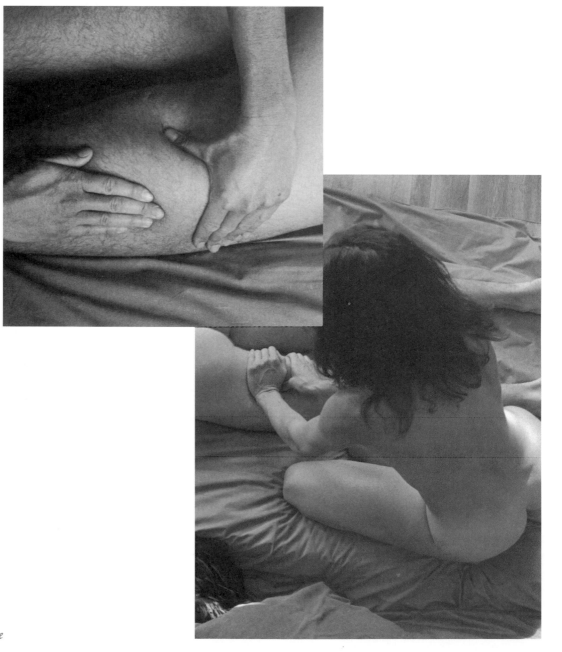

Generally, friction strokes will reach through the skin to massage the underlying muscles; a very light variation is reserved for stimulating the skin itself. On the penetrating strokes, press down until you feel solid muscular tissue. Avoid surface blood vessels and bony parts of the body like the ribs. Use one hand to steady the body — your "anchor hand" — the other to apply friction. Lean forward to put weight on your hands and rotate your fingertips on the muscles, not the skin.

Friction travels easily. By moving your hands up and down the body as you rotate your fingers, you can easily cover an entire muscle group — such as the trapezius on the top of the back or the hamstrings on the back of the thigh — in a few minutes. Friction promotes blood circulation deep within the body and aids lymph flow. It's especially effective over major joints like the shoulder and hip where other massage movements are difficult. Just minutes after you begin, your partner feels an irresistible penetrating warmth. Nothing you can do during massage makes things happen faster than friction.

Friction aids the fluid release effect by applying direct pressure to interior tissues that other strokes cannot always reach.

◆ Spot Friction: Sore muscles crave spot friction. Focus on one spot and stay there until your partner feels better. Your anchor hand continuously pushes flesh toward the friction hand.
◆ Fingertip Friction: Your fingertips fit where the hands can't go: in the crevices of the hand and foot and around the sides of the eyes and mouth. Steady your partner with your anchor hand. Pressures vary from heavy on the foot to light on most parts of the hands and face.

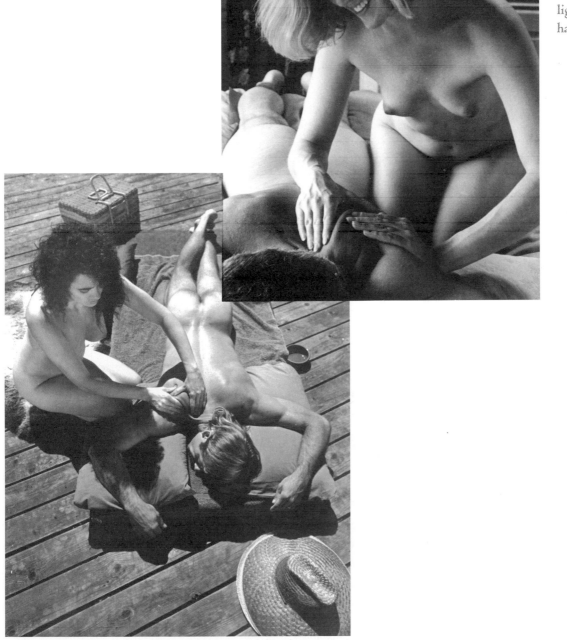

Percussion

Percussion takes massage where it normally cannot go: beneath the ribs to the body's vital organs and deep within the limbs to the bones themselves. Get it right and you will set up irresistible waves of vibration that carry right through the entire body. You don't need oil to do percussion. Start with these strokes when massaging highly stressed individuals. Percussion gives your partner an excuse to relax and surrender to the experience. Newcomers to massage sometimes find percussion off-putting because the rapid "blows" look as though they could be painful. Executed properly, however, the "blows" become a light tapping — a gentle rain, not a thunderstorm.

Concentrate on visible muscles when you do percussion. Stay off surface blood vessels and bony structures, especially the spine. Every percussion stroke must be cushioned either by snapping your wrists just before your hand makes contact with your partner's body or, on the more intense strokes, striking the back of your own hand. Get feedback from your partner on pressures that feel good; preferences vary greatly. Select a comfortable speed that you will be able to maintain for several minutes, if need be. Percussion is like riding a bicycle: You can continue for long periods if you don't rush it.

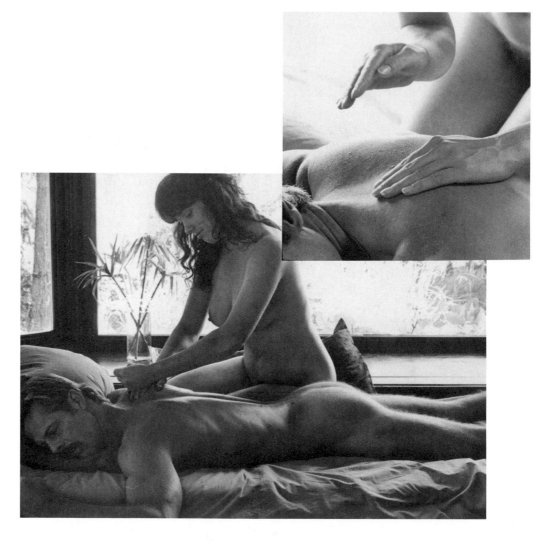

Percussion speeds the fluid release effect by stirring up accumulated acidic wastes deep within the body. Athletes and heavily muscled types cannot seem to get enough back percussion. Combined with kneading and friction, percussion strokes provide the perfect sequence for relieving fatigued muscles in the upper back, and around the neck and shoulders. A two- or three-stroke sequence works wonders on the long muscles that run parallel to the spine.

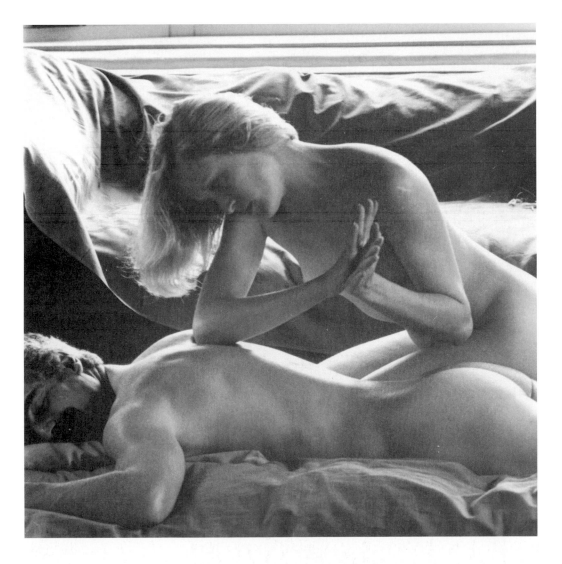

♦ Before you "throw" an arm or leg, move it back and forth slowly to test for the point of tension. Catch the limb well inside of the spot where you felt resistance. Set limits to your passive exercises and stay with them.

The more deliberate and informed your touch becomes during massage, the more trust you will build.

Passive Exercise

You do all the work; your partner need only experience the massage during passive exercise sequences. You might want to remind her of that before you begin lest she be tempted to help you lift a limb or rotate a joint. Some of the most exquisitely sensual moments in massage involve simple antigravity effects: while a part of your partner's body floats through the air, she does nothing at all. Yes, you can rotate your own joints, fling your arms through the air, and arch your back, but what a difference to have it done for you.

Passive exercises increase the body's mobility. Unconsciously, we train the body to work within limitations. As we accept stiffness, our muscles begin to move in shorter arcs. Passive exercise reverses this training. Buried deep within the joints and inaccessible to ordinary massage, tiny ligaments that hold bones together are stretched gently. Tendons are extended to the point of resistance several times and then slightly beyond. Production of

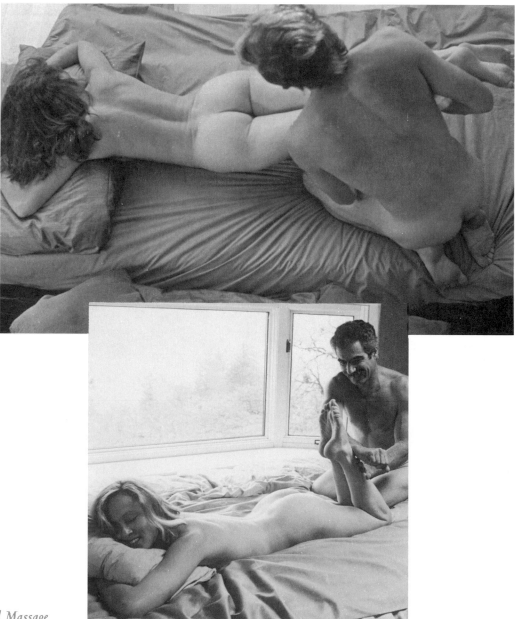

synovial fluid, the internal joint lubricant, is stimulated. Afterwards, chronic stiffness disappears; the whole body seems more supple and fluid.

The human body was designed, whether by evolution or accident, to make these strokes easy to do. Every time you begin a lift, you will discover a natural handle — at the wrists, ankles, chin, shoulders, and lower back — waiting. Take hold of these handy projections, which are identified throughout the book, at the start of each passive exercise movement.

Performed separately or combined with other strokes, passive exercises are great favorites during group massage sessions (see pages 164–65). Two limbs float through the air at once — three, four. Hands bob and roll, fingers flutter. Parts of the body take off and fly while large muscles are kneaded into deep relaxation elsewhere. Again, you cannot experience this mix of sensations outside of massage.

There is something primal and infinitely tender in the full-body passive exercises. Your partner is lifted into the air and gently lowered, held and carried, perhaps for the first time since childhood.

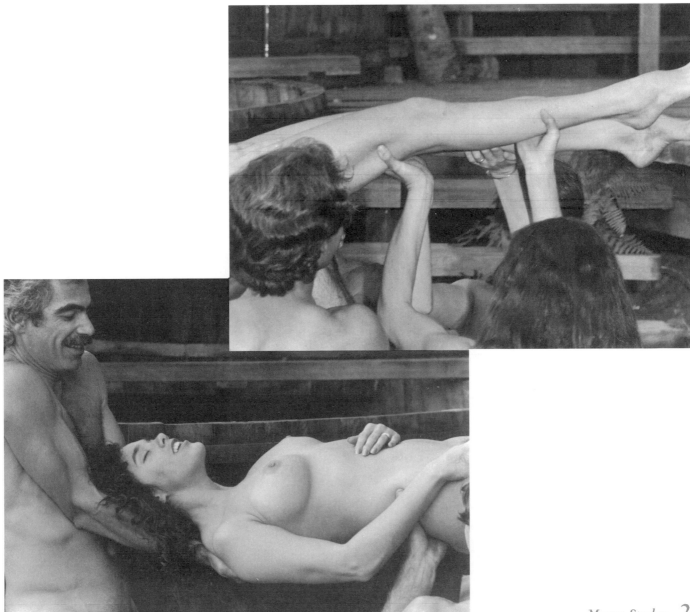

Compression

Compression gives you a chance to rest for a moment while maintaining meaningful contact with your partner. It's the easiest massage stroke — you'll get it right the first time you try.

First, make yourself comfortable so you're not reaching too far to the left or right. You may want to sit back on a pillow during this leisurely stroke. Since your hands do not move in the full rest position, called passive compression, you don't need oil. Press down on a broad part of the body like the forehead, the back of the knee or the base of the spine, making contact from the fingertips to the base of your palm. Let your contact hand mold itself to the shape of your partner's body; your fingertips should trace the contour of every curve.

Oil generously before active compression. Circle on muscular parts of the body with one or two hands, while pressing down firmly. On large body areas make contact with the full surface of your hand. Use the flat part of your knuckles (as shown) to do compression on the thick tendons around the larger joints. Press down into the muscle tissue and circle slowly, three times in each direction.

Use compression when you're not sure what to do next. It's welcome everywhere on the body, and the good feelings that follow build confidence in your ability as a masseur.

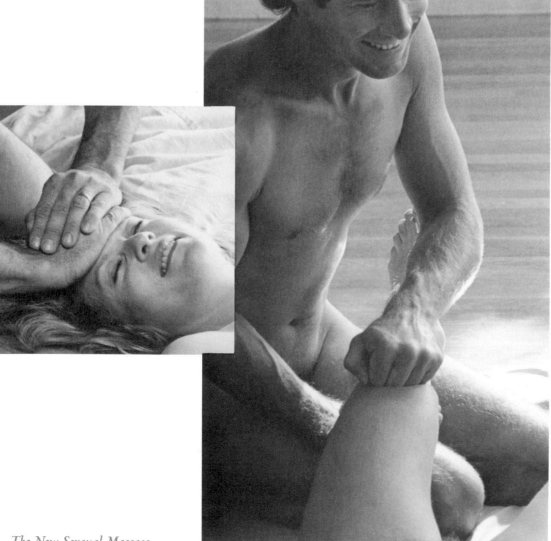

PART 2

A Complete Body Massage

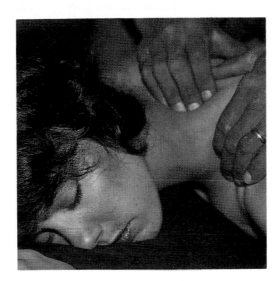

CHAPTER 4

The Back

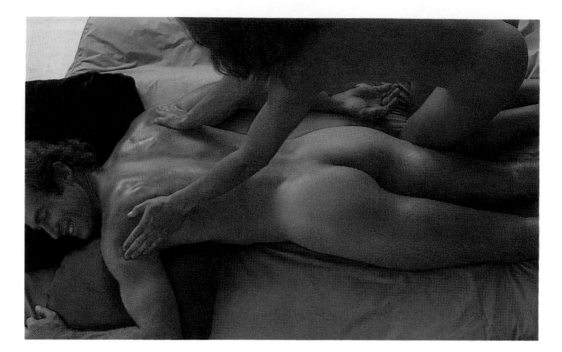

The way to get to paradise is to go there. As a masseur, you are the vehicle; all the better if it's your partner's first massage — you're going to take him on a trip he will never forget.

If you want to relax the whole body, there is no better place to begin than the back. Since we use the back in nearly everything we do, tension tends to accumulate in the larger muscles, especially those near the spine, the body's switchboard. Sensation from the fingertips to the toes is routed through large spinal nerves on the way to the brain. Drain stress from the long vertical muscles that run parallel to the spine and virtually every stroke you do elsewhere on the body will be more effective. By relaxing the back first, you will increase your partner's enjoyment throughout the massage.

If it's a first massage and your partner is shy about being touched (but may secretly crave it), a few minutes of back massage provides an ideal icebreaker. Good back massage brings a sense of consummate relief followed by deep waves of sensual pleasure, a mood change so profound that people simply melt and surrender to the feeling.

*B*ack massage also gives you a chance to learn a bit about the body you're massaging. Ask for feedback now because a few strokes into the massage your partner will be too relaxed to talk. The back will accept more pressure than other parts of the body — determine the upper limit here. Choose a rhythm that will feel good throughout the massage and stay with it. Big strokes and little strokes should be done at the same pace. Now is the time to find out what rhythm suits your partner. But be sure not to start an involved conversation that will distract both of you. A few words will do.

Your partner rarely experiences tension as a purely mental state; she doesn't simply *feel* tense, some part of her body actually *is* tense. Locating and relaxing the specific muscles that cause tension make the mind-body connection work for you during massage.

One of the most crucial relationships between muscle tension and stress becomes apparent when you massage the long muscles that run parallel to the spine. Pressure on the spine pulls directly on the nervous system's fibrous core, causing tension to shoot out in all directions. As nearby muscles become rigid, pressure on the spine increases. You can break this vicious circle of stress with circulation and fingertip kneading sequences. Relax the muscles around the spine and every other stroke you do will be more effective. Sometimes, after a half dozen or so particularly satisfying strokes, your partner will sigh gratefully, but don't expect an audible confirmation for everything you do. Relaxation is a deeply personal experience — your thanks will come later.

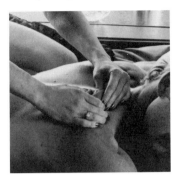
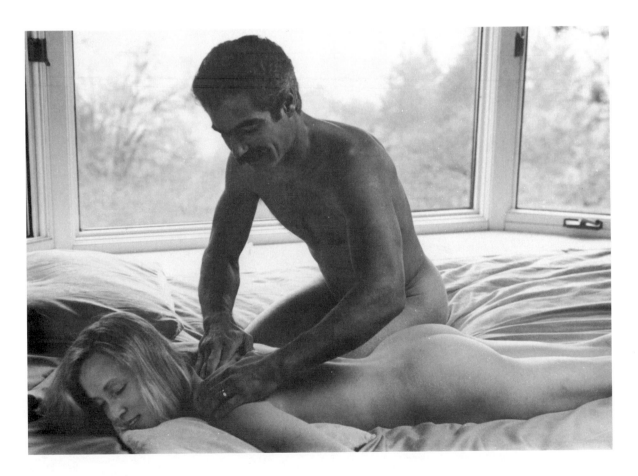

Initially, your partner may lie down with his hands over his head, a position that's only temporarily comfortable. Eventually, if the shoulder blades remain elevated and unsupported, the muscles of the upper back will become tense. If your partner lies down in this position, try suggesting (never give orders during massage) that he might be more comfortable with his hands by his sides. Begin to lift one arm as you make the suggestion so he will understand that he's not expected to do anything. With one hand above and one hand below your partner's elbow, lift the arms, one at a time. Move his arms about six inches away from his body. If he prefers to keep his arms up, slip a small pillow under each shoulder for extra support. Pillows provide quick support beneath the knees, ankles, neck, lower back, and other parts of the body — have a few on hand when you do massage.

It's helpful to divide the back into three areas before you begin: the muscles that run parallel to the spine, the top, and the sides. Your back massage will focus on each one of these areas in turn.

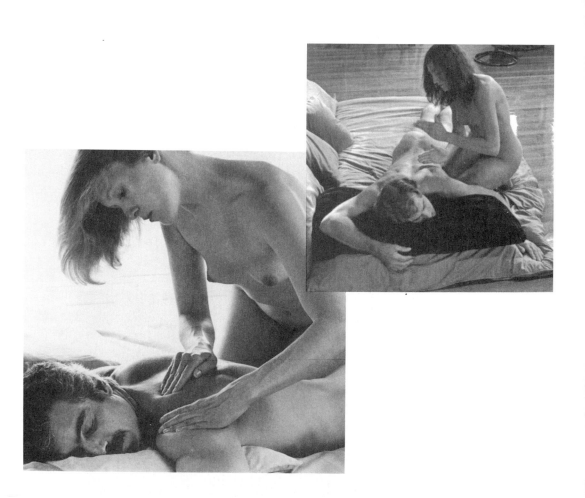

Hand-Over-Hand Pulling

Begin massage with a stroke that lets your partner get used to the feeling of your hands moving across his body. Starting from his neck, work down the back with a simple hand-over-hand pulling motion. Keep your fingers together and your thumbs flat. Use your thumbs to define the inside border of the stroke, tracing the raised muscles that run parallel to the spine from the neck to the waist. Stay off the spine itself. Keep the full surface of your hands in contact with your partner's back throughout (as shown). Apply even pressure from your fingertips to the base of your palm.

Begin with one hand at the bottom of the back in the palms-down starting position you used for the first movement. Put your other hand in the same position on the other side of the spine but at the top of your partner's back. Your lower hand remains still and in contact while your upper hand pulls down from neck to hip. When you reach the hips with one hand, leave it stationary and lift the other, placing it on the top of the back. Then begin moving down from the neck while pressing down with the second hand. Don't be afraid to use plenty of pressure. By this time you may begin to notice a tangible difference in the way your partner's back feels. Muscles are beginning to soften as you pump oxygen into the tissues and squeeze out wastes. The fluid release effect has begun.

OILING

♦ Put your oil container midway between your partner's waist and shoulders, where you can reach it easily. Keep a large towel nearby. Remember to add oil to your own hands, then spread it across the area you're about to massage. Never pour oil directly onto your partner's body. Don't interrupt a stroke if you discover a speck of grit on the skin. Remove it with one hand while continuing to massage with the other.

Spread oil across the whole surface of the back and onto the shoulders and sides. Oiling the back marks the beginning of your full-body massage. Whenever possible, blend oiling with individual massage strokes. Stay in contact with your partner while you oil.

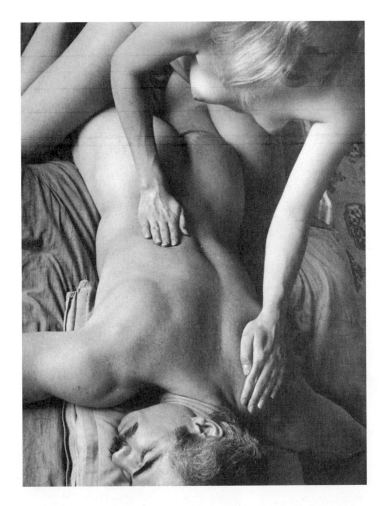

Back Circulation

First, oil from the waist to the shoulder tops, making sure to include the sides of the back. Add oil to your hands — never pour it directly onto your partner's back — and spread it liberally in wide flat-hand strokes. Use extra oil if your partner has a hairy back. Oiling here marks your first contact with your partner's body, an important moment. Don't break contact until the end of the massage.

Resting your knees on a small pillow, kneel alongside your partner's waist or, for better balance, straddle him (as shown). Make contact from the tips of your fingers to the base of your palms. With the base of your palms at your partner's hips, flatten out your hands so his spine will pass between your thumbs. Rest the base of your palms against the two muscular ridges that run parallel to the spine. While avoiding pressing on the spine itself, press up the back on these long muscles. Use plenty of pressure — these are powerful muscles. Push forward, molding your

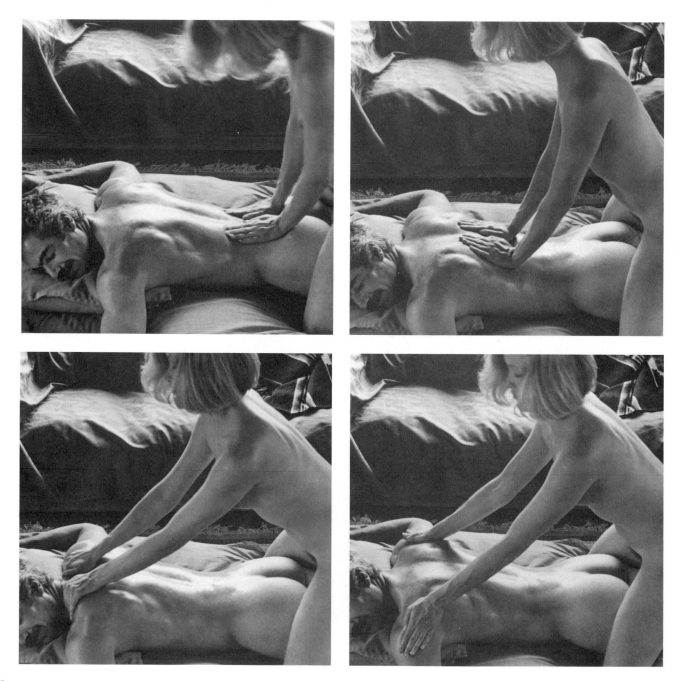

hands to the changing shape of your partner's body. Lean forward with your whole body as you stroke, especially between the shoulder blades.

When you reach the neck, turn your hands so they slide across your partner's shoulders out to the top of the arm. Then, turn your hands again and begin moving down his back. Avoid one of the most common mistakes in massage, permitting a part of your hand to break contact unnecessarily. Be sure you can feel his side from the base of your palm to your fingertips.

Pull your hands all the way down your partner's sides until they reach the flared part of his hips. Then, turn slowly and return to the bottom of the spine where you began. Each of your turns at the bottom and top of the back should be executed smoothly, without hesitation, so that what your partner feels is one long, continuous motion from the base of his spine over the shoulders, down his sides, and across the top of his hips.

Quite often, the first concrete sign you have that this stroke is working is a series of long, hearty sighs from your partner. This means he's beginning to unwind and would enjoy more of the same. Be generous — give him what he wants.

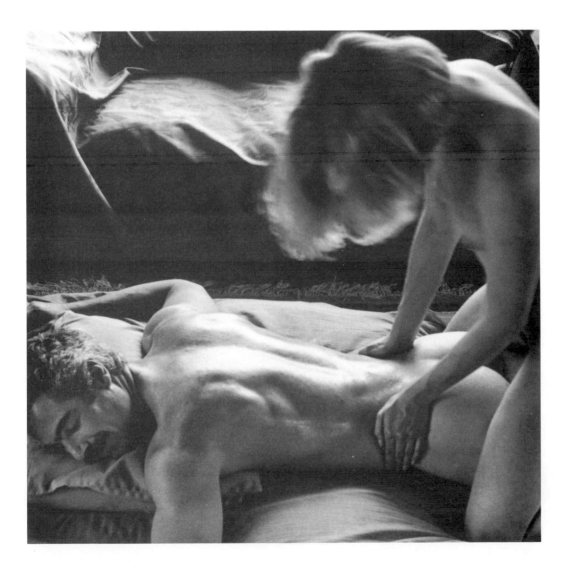

"People are so accustomed to thinking of the body as an instrument or a tool of the mind that they accept its relative deadness as a normal state. They measure bodies in pounds and inches and compare their shape with idealized forms, completely ignoring the fact that what is important is how the body feels.

"The discovery that the body has a life of its own and the capacity to heal itself is a revelation of hope."

Alexander Lowen, M.D., *The Betrayal of the Body* (Ontario: Collier-Macmillan Canada Ltd., 1967), p. 209.

Back Compression

Important as the muscles along the spine are, by now the rest of your partner's back will be begging for attention. Move away from the spine with compression, an easy-to-learn stroke that will focus your massage on almost any part of the back. The following compression sequence will cover the whole back from a single massage position at your partner's side. Don't hesitate to linger over obviously tense areas. Simply repeat compression over hardened muscles until you feel them yield.

Keeping one hand in contact with your partner's back, move over so you're sitting alongside him. Put one hand against his back with your fingers extended and touching. Your fingertips should touch the muscles that run parallel to the spine (but stay off the spine itself) while the base of your palm contacts the edge of his back. Now put your other hand on top of the first hand in exactly the same position (as shown). Start near the shoulders. With your hands resting on top of each other, press down and begin to turn in small circles. Move down the back slowly. Press down on the heel of your hands over the larger muscle groups.

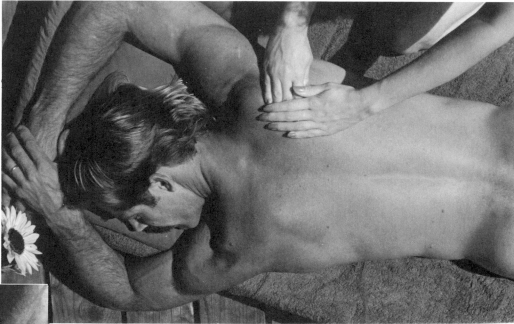

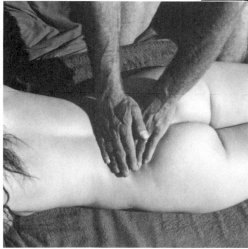

When you reach your partner's hips, cross over the spine very lightly (as shown) applying pressure with your fingertips and go up the other side of the back.

Stick to a slow, easy rhythm while you circle and don't worry if you can't reach all the way over to your partner's opposite side. Go as far as you can comfortably — you can always sit on the other side of his body while you circle on that side of the back. Circle the back three times, rotating your hands slowly.

When massaging difficult-to-reach muscle groups (or with large hands on a small partner), use only your fingertips. Fingertip kneading, friction, and percussion movements allow you to spread the benefits of massage to the body's tiniest surfaces. During compression, apply pressure to your fingertips by turning your hands at sharp angles to each other (as shown). The powerful trapezius muscle wraps around the back of the neck where full-hand strokes are difficult. Reach behind the neck with your fingertips to massage it.

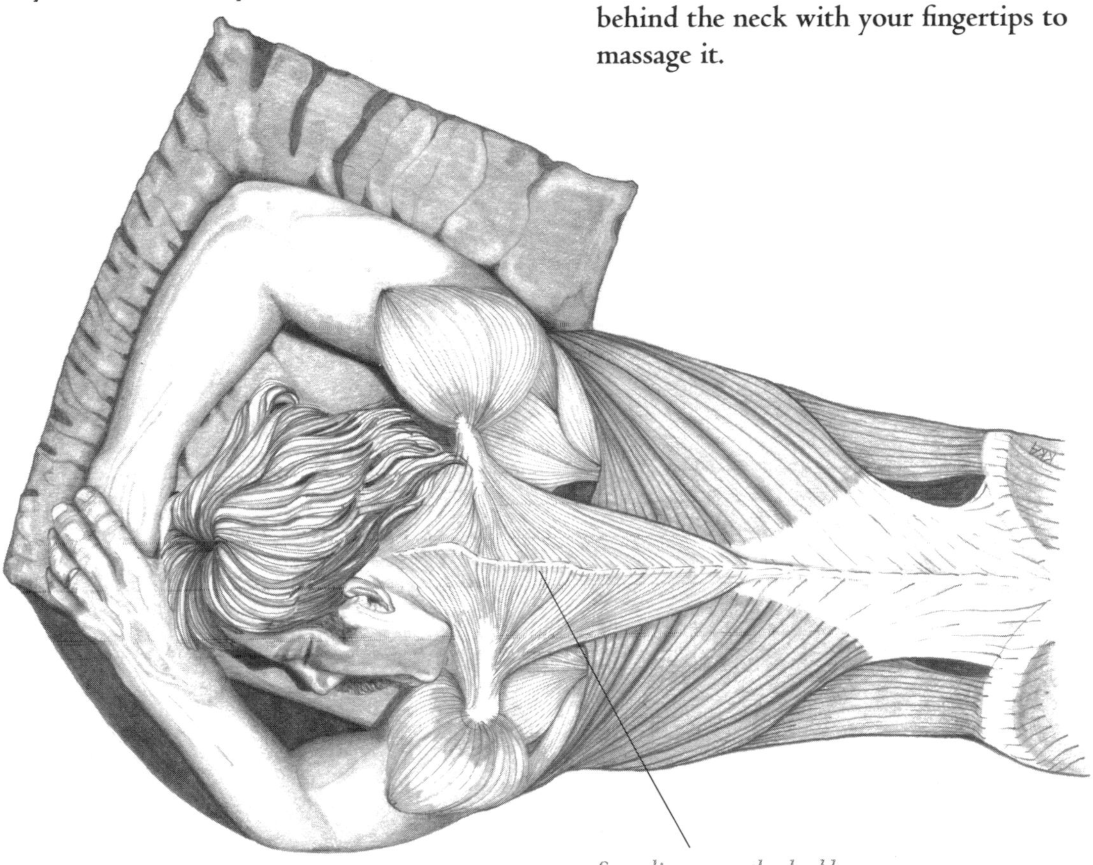

Spreading across the shoulders and down the middle of the back, the massive trapezius muscle helps support the head. Relax this muscle first if your partner suffers from stiff neck and headache pain.

THE SOURCE OF HEADACHES

♦ Masseurs view many supposedly psychological problems as purely physical phenomenon. Go directly to the body and you can create mood changes that last for hours, even days. Your partner's headache, for example, is hardly "all in her head." The head is a heavy object that must be carried throughout the day.

Twisting, turning, and stretching constantly, the massive trapezius (shown below) does most of the work. A tensed trapezius puts direct pressure on nerves just beneath the shoulder blades, which are closely tied to stress headaches. If your partner has been suffering from a stiff neck or tension headaches, give extra attention to this muscle during your back massage. Relax the trapezius now and your head massage will be far more effective.

Spot Friction

If your partner complained about a specific ache before you began, try a minute or two of spot friction, a basic rubbing movement that can be directed anywhere on the back. You needn't add oil to do this stroke. In fact, friction will work on a perfectly dry skin. Women generally carry tension around the neck and shoulders while men usually experience soreness due to muscle fatigue in the lower back. Let your partner show you where it hurts.

Then, press down a few inches away from the sore spot with one hand, holding your fingers together and thumb wide open. This hand is called the "anchor hand" and you will use it to gather up loose flesh while pressing in to the open space between your forefinger and thumb. Once you have your anchor hand in place pushing up a generous roll of flesh, you're ready to press down on the sore spot itself with all four fingers of your other hand. Circle slowly while you press down. In friction strokes, your hand doesn't move across the skin but rather circles on the muscle tissue below. Avoid pulling on your

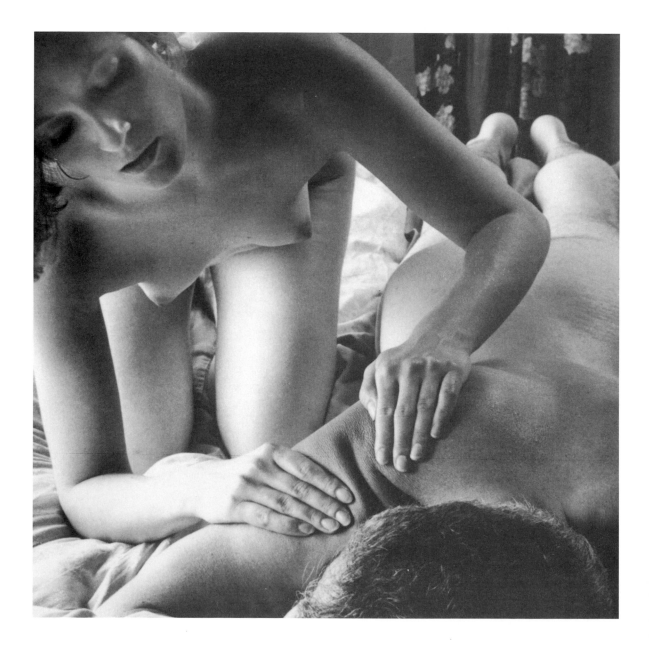

partner's skin while you circle. Press folds of loose flesh toward the sore area repeatedly with your anchor hand.

Like every stroke in this book, friction feels good whether or not your partner has sore muscles. If you manage to locate hidden soreness, spend extra time on those spots. Friction strokes, unlike drugs, can vanquish specific pains caused by fatigued muscles without knocking out the whole central nervous system.

Ask her where it hurts. Then, move in with friction until she feels no pain.

♦ As your partner begins to focus on pure feeling, your hands enter into a kind of silent dialogue with his body. You can feel him following your touch, noting everything that you do. Watch for the secret smiles. Listen. His very breathing signifies pleasure. This is real massage, one of the most ancient human relationships.

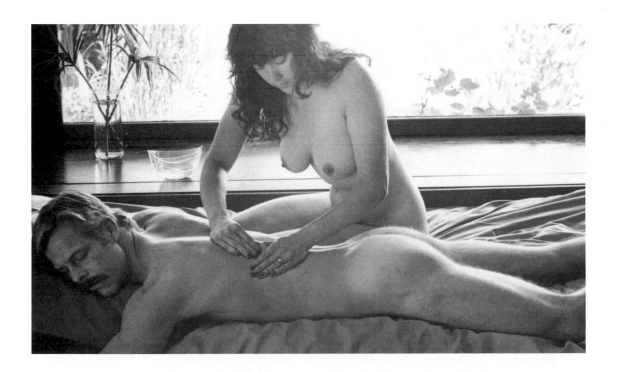

The Forearm Press

If you're massaging someone with a large back, it's fun to circle with your whole forearm. Your partner feels an interesting new texture and big things happen across the whole back. Oil your forearm thoroughly and hold it midway between the hand and elbow (as shown). Pressing down firmly, circle slowly. Bending your hand forward makes additional contact with your knuckle and the heel of your hand possible. Look for the thickest muscles, the fleshiest tissues. Move up and down your partner's back with your forearm and, of course, go easy when you cross the spine.

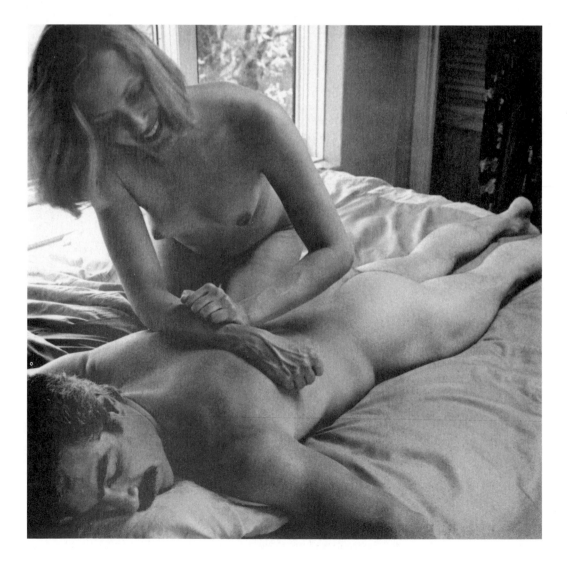

Kneading the Shoulders

Knead the back from the top down, starting on the shoulders. This is an ideal place to practice kneading because the shoulders and the back of the neck almost always need extra attention. Learn to work around bony spots and focus on powerful muscles that support the head. Kneading travels easily — most of the fleshy tissue between the shoulders is ideal for the grasping and squeezing part of the stroke. Expect to knead across the top of the back a dozen or more times, when learning. Your partner will enjoy the extra attention.

The basic kneading movement described on page 17 will adapt easily to the changing texture of your partner's body. Use your thumb to pick up folds of flesh and remember to keep your other fingers together. Whether focusing on a single tight spot on the back of the neck or traveling across your partner's body, move your hands in regular circles. One hand picks up a fold of flesh while the other opens wide at the thumb and forefinger. Use your whole hand on fleshy areas. As you approach bony structures like the shoulder blades, knead with your fingertips. Big strokes move at the same speed as little strokes.

Knead the back of the neck while your partner's head is turned to one side. Here again, concentrate, with your fingertips, on the thick muscular base of the neck; it will never be easier to reach. You will see tiny folds of flesh rise with your circling hands. Then you will feel a tangible softening as tensed muscles begin to relax.

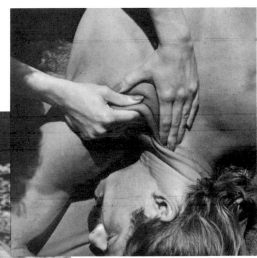

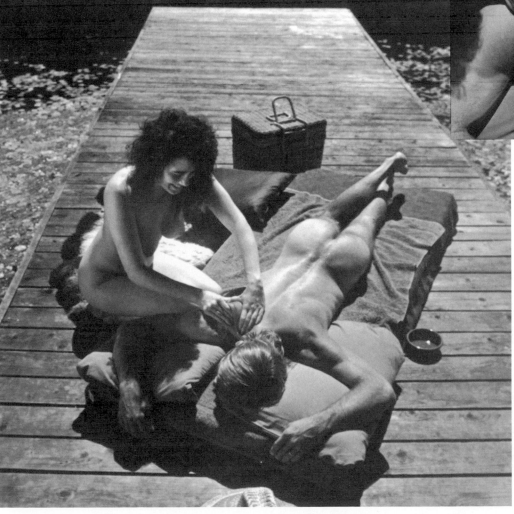

Fingertip Kneading
the Back

Kneading strokes travel so naturally that you often cannot resist wandering onto a nearby area before you're through. The long muscles that run parallel to the spine, recently relaxed by your massive circulation stroke, stand ready to be kneaded. They fit nicely between your fingertips. Move up and down each side of the spine three times, reversing direction at the neck and hips. Avoid pressing against the spine. While kneading, you should feel muscle and flesh, never bone, beneath your fingertips.

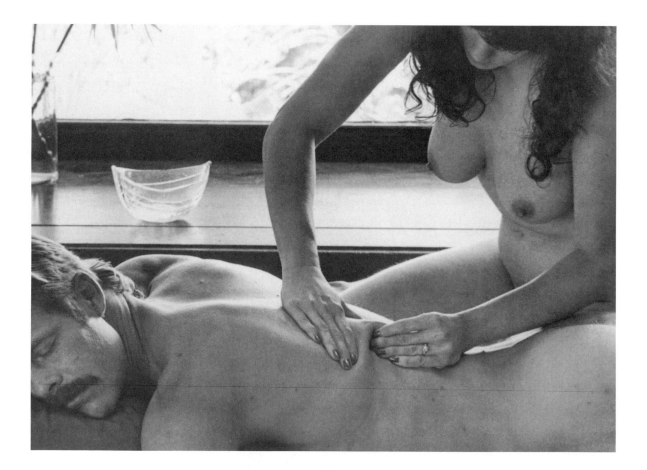

Knuckle Pressing

Good massage requires technique, not strength. If your partner craves more pressure, use your own body weight to focus a penetrating stroke on the thick muscles of his back.

Grasp your hand at the wrist (as shown) and press the flat part of your knuckles against his back. Rotate your knuckle on the fleshiest tissues but avoid pressing down beneath his ribs where the top of the kidney is exposed. A few minutes of knuckle pressing feels wonderful on tensed shoulder muscles — but don't stop there. Move up and down the back from the shoulders to the hips on both sides of the spine.

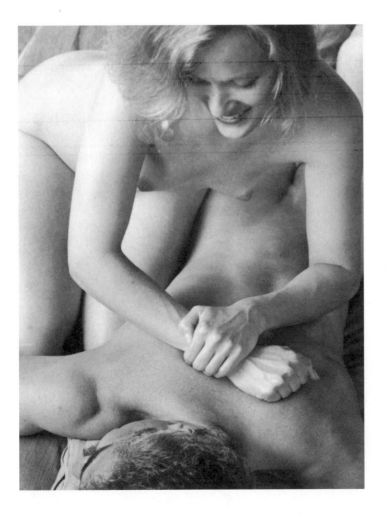

♦ Perhaps when we started describing ourselves as "stressed" instead of merely nervous (which seemed temporary), we were conceding, permanently, our ability to relax. If we pursue relaxation as though it were a career goal — adding more activities in order to slow down — tension becomes a permanent fact of life. When the pills, therapies, and exercise programs fail, what's left?

If you've been working through this book with a friend, you know the answer. You want to shout: For heaven's sake, *get a massage.* But shouting at stressed people only makes them tense. Give your partner a massage instead of an argument.

In fact, give him a back massage. Everyone secretly craves a long, infinitely relaxing back massage. Think of it as the supreme icebreaker, the best possible way to demonstrate the power of massage. Do it now, if you aren't already doing it.

Forearm Spread

Be sure you've oiled the whole back before you begin this luxurious movement.

No matter how much technique you master, your hands can cover only a small part of the back at any moment. To satisfy your partner's desire for more contact, use your forearms (again, instead of your hands) to blanket the whole back with deep sensation. Start with your forearms pressed tightly together at the center of your partner's back and spread them slowly to the far limits of your reach. Making a fist with both hands, bend forward at the wrist to make knuckle contact along the side of the body. Keep your arms extended straight ahead while you move back and forth across the back.

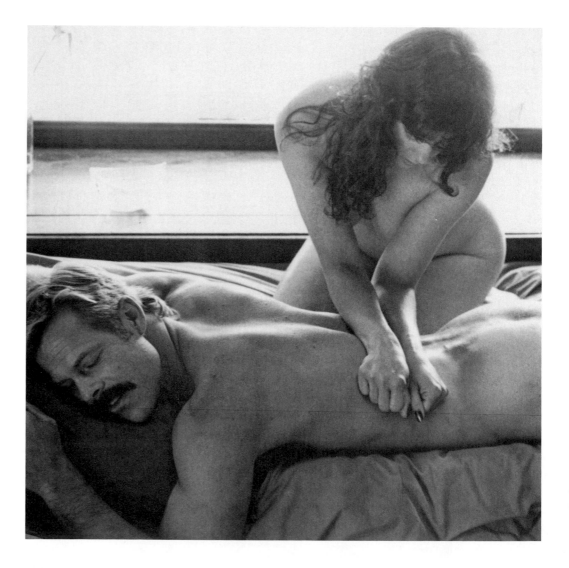

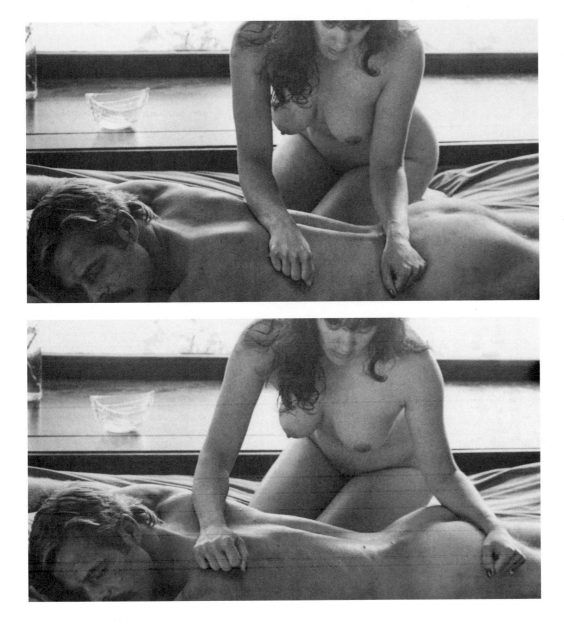

A thorough back massage should include nearby muscles that exert pressure on the back as well as those that extend from the back to other parts of the body. The large latissimus dorsi wraps around the side of the body to support the arms. Bend your hands at the wrist to massage it during the forearm spread. Add a full-hand kneading stroke, like the one you used on the shoulders, to reach down to the gluteus maximus just below the hip. Knead the side of your partner's body from the top of the leg to the arms, and back.

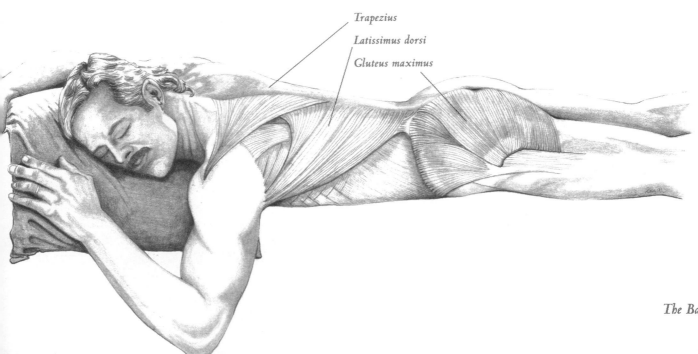

Trapezius

Latissimus dorsi

Gluteus maximus

The Back **43**

Rolling the Back

When you relax the muscles along the spine and at the shoulders, the surface tissues of the back become more supple. This is a tangible sign of your partner's mood. He's melting.

Now you can actually pick up folds of skin and roll them between your thumb and four fingers (as shown). Start at the bottom of the spine and work up to the neck. Push a fold of flesh forward with your thumb and, while grasping it with your fingers, pull straight up with your thumb.

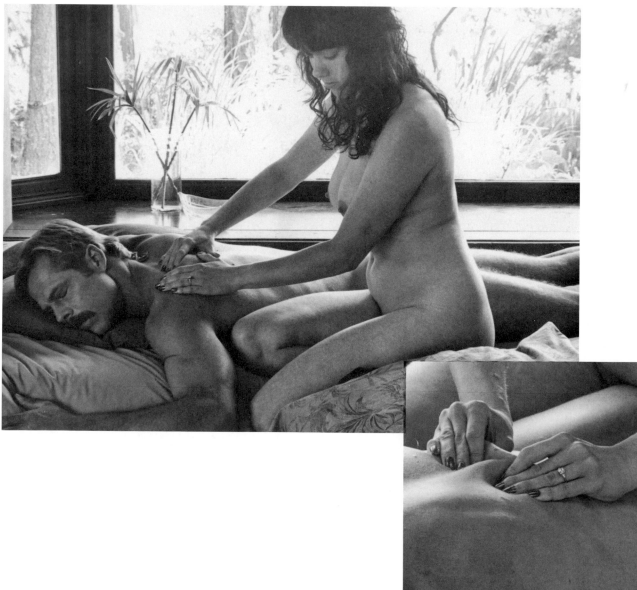

Headaches and the Scapula Lift

Much of the tension that headache sufferers experience actually originates in the upper back and neck. Feel the muscles along the shoulder blade. Important nerves that supply the head originate beneath the bony scapula. As long as tensed muscles press down on the nerves that supply the head, your partner's headache will rage on. Before he reaches for a drug that will numb the entire central nervous system and strain the kidneys, try this simple massage sequence that goes directly to the hidden source of tension headaches.

Relax the neck and upper back in three stages. First, fingertip knead back and forth across the shoulders, lingering on the thickly muscled back of the neck. While kneading, you will get a good sense of various tight spots where tension has accumulated. Return to each one with a penetrating spot friction movement. Finally, cup one hand over the back of the shoulder blade while lifting from directly below the same spot on the front of your partner's body (as shown). Rotate the whole shoulder blade as you lift. Support builds trust. The more secure your partner feels, the quicker he will yield to the effects of this stroke. Rotate the shoulder blade three times in each direction. At the end of the final rotation, reach beneath the shoulder blade with your fingertips (as shown) to apply friction to the hidden source of so many tension headaches. Lift at the elbow if you decide to reach across your partner's body. From that position, however, you cannot rotate the shoulder blade as you lift.

◆ Press down on the muscles around the shoulder blades with your fingertips. Do they feel tight and

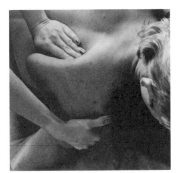

lumpy? Important nerves that supply the head originate beneath the shoulder blades. Tensed muscles here will keep the whole area tight as a drum, a condition that you can easily feel. Until all pressure on the nerves is relieved, your partner's headache will rage on.

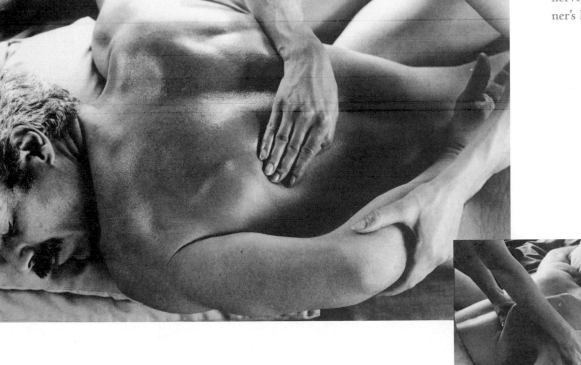

Massaging the Heart and Lungs

To reach interior tissues on the arms and legs you need only press down a bit harder while massaging. But since the rib cage, the body's largest bony structure, lies just beneath the back, ordinary massage strokes cannot penetrate much beyond the muscular surface. To massage the heart, lungs, and other vital organs, use percussion strokes that carry right through the entire body.

The effect of a few minutes of percussion on internal organs, particularly the lungs where oxygen enters the blood, could hardly be more dramatic. In a matter of seconds, acidic wastes, nerve debris, and pollutants in the lungs are shaken loose and later expelled from the body. At the same time, blood oxygen levels soar throughout the body, leaving your partner feeling refreshed and invigorated.

Percussion movements can be done one at a time but they work best as a family of related strokes. Each one transmits slightly different waves of sensation all the way through the torso. A simple wrist movement absorbs most of the downward energy of the stroke; instead of a "blow" you deliver a light tapping sensation which gently shakes the vital organs. Rather than a specific point of impact, your partner feels a general vibration. Percussion also works its magic on the muscular surface tissues of the back where knotted muscles that refuse to yield to other strokes finally begin to relax.

Nobody can resist a few minutes of mixed percussion. Often the turning point in a full-body massage, particularly when massaging tensed individuals, these strokes prove the power of massage. And when you stop, your partner goes on vibrating silently.

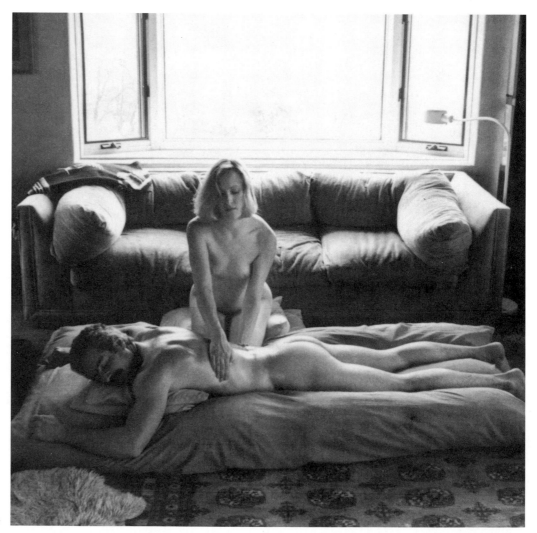

Thumping the Back

If your partner is tense, his thoughts are elsewhere. You need a breakthrough stroke to awaken the body and put massage center stage. Back thumping gets their attention every time.

Every percussion movement must be cushioned to absorb excessive pressure. This stroke combines two of the most common cushioning techniques: striking the back of your anchor hand, instead of making direct contact with your partner's body, and breaking the stroke at the wrist just before you make contact.

Back thumping travels effortlessly. Make a fist with one hand — your percussion hand — and mold the fingers of the other hand — your anchor hand — to the area you wish to massage. Begin striking the back of your anchor hand's fingers with the side of your percussion hand (as shown). Break the stroke at the wrist just before you make contact.

Move across the shoulders and up and down the long rows of muscles that run parallel to the spine. But stay off the spine itself and other bony structures.

◆ Consider the percussion strokes that follow and the great half-body lift, which requires a degree of muscle power, as optional during

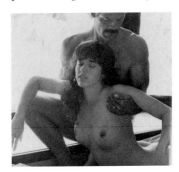

a full-body massage. They create a bright, stimulating mood, a counterpoint to the feeling of naked hands gliding across oiled skin. Use percussion to awaken an overstressed "deadened" body. Athletes with muscular backs enjoy the dynamic "clear" feeling afterward — so do headache sufferers. A few minutes of vigorous percussion invigorates your partner and leaves the torso feeling alive and tingling.

If, however, your partner has already entered a sensual reverie, sighing as muscles relax and moaning with pleasure from time to time, you may not want to interrupt the mood. Move on to the full-body stroke on page 51 and save percussion for your next massage.

The Back **47**

◆ Too much pressure causes tight muscles to contract further — leaving your partner's body less relaxed at the end of the massage than at the beginning. Chronic muscle tension forms a kind of shield, a body armor, that comes between your partner and his feelings. But tense bodies have the same capacity for sensuality as relaxed ones. By relaxing perpetually tensed muscles, massage makes lasting relaxation possible.

Elbow Pounding

Outside of the chest and back lifts — mere icing on your massage cake — few strokes require extra physical strength. Even the percussion movements, which must penetrate to interior tissues, work best with light to moderate pressures.

When percussion breaks through body armor — and it will — your partner's first request will probably be for more pressure. Increase pressure slowly, resisting the temptation to bear down hard; he may really want more repetition. By plunging on heedlessly with deep percussion, you risk a descent into mindless back beating. The moment pleasure turns to pain, you've sacrificed the whole massage.

With that caveat, you may want to try elbow pounding on heavily muscled types who crave truly penetrating sensations.

The extra leverage created by your whole forearm permits you to increase pressure no matter what the size relationship between you and your partner. And it involves a new part of your body, the elbow, in the massage. Your partner will enjoy the interesting shape and the way the tip of your elbow fits perfectly over the long muscles that run parallel to his spine.

While slowly moving your elbow up and down the spinal muscles and across the top of the back, strike the open palm of your hand. Control the stroke with your contact arm, bringing more pressure to bear on heavily muscled tissues, less on softer areas.

You get back what you give in massage. How long has it been since someone appreciated your elbow?

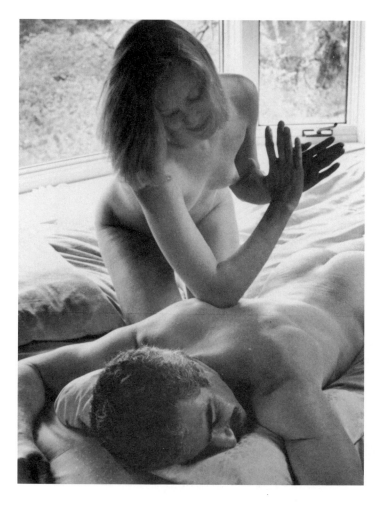

Cupping

Listen again during cupping, the loudest percussion stroke. Bend your hands to form an upside-down cup and bring them down one after another on your partner's back. This time you'll hear a crisp popping sound every time your fingers meet flesh. The more air you trap under the cupped part of your hands, the louder the popping becomes. Be sure to break each downward stroke at the wrist.

Move up and down the thickly muscled parts of the back and back and forth across the shoulders. Remember, stay off the spine itself.

Use cupping to wake up a sluggish, unfeeling body, but go easy on this stroke during a full-body massage. This movement builds an intensity of its own, particularly when used for an extended period on the back to control stress. Cupping once or twice around the back warms the muscles and awakens the nerves; much more than that can overstimulate your partner.

The Pinky Snap

This stroke permits you to focus percussion on a tiny area, like the base of the neck, where full-hand massage becomes difficult. It also feels good on larger muscle groups but the penetrating effect there is reduced. Serve it up as a dessert after a main course of deep percussion.

Keeping your hands close enough for the palms to brush, bring the sides of your fingers, one hand at a time, down onto your partner's back (as shown). Your pinkies should hang down to absorb the force of the stroke, contacting the back one hand at a time. Speed is less important than consistent rhythm.

Listen. When you hear a soft rhythmic clicking, you've got it just right.

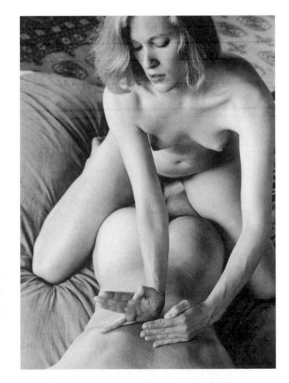

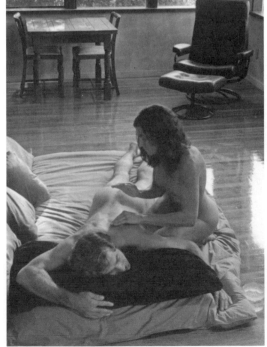

The Back Lift

Raising the shoulders, one of the body's most convenient natural handles, allows you to flex your partner's lower back, a notorious tension trap. The back lift creates another one of those delightful feelings that simply cannot be duplicated outside of massage: While the top half of your partner's body rises into the air, the bottom half relaxes on the massage surface.

Reach under the armpits and clasp your hands behind the neck. For balance during the lift, bring your knee up and put one foot flat on the floor. Rhythm is even more important during lifts than the rest of massage. Avoid sharp, jerky movements, lest you lose the trust you've been building. Your partner's body should rise and fall effortlessly. Lift slowly to the point of tension, then hold for a few moments and lower your partner to the massage surface. As the back begins to feel more supple, rotate it a bit from side to side when you reach the top of the lift.

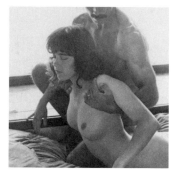

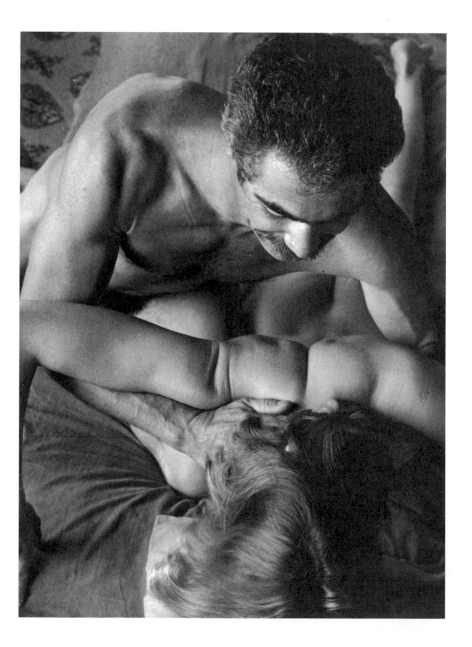

Full-Body Circulation

This single luxurious circulation stroke spreads deepening waves of pleasure from one end of the body to the other. It's the perfect way to move from the back to the next part of your full-body massage, the back of the legs.

Transitions are tactile events in massage — never break contact. If your hands lead the way, your partner will follow the sensation as it moves from one part of the body to another.

Move down the outer thigh, pulling toward your partner's feet with all four fingers while cupping the back of the legs with your thumbs. Kneel at the feet and cup your hands over your partner's ankles (as shown). Before starting, glance at the spot next to your partner's waist. You will probably need to reposition yourself (as shown on next page) at least once during this stroke so make sure you have a soft surface, perhaps a pillow, for your knees and a convenient place for your oil.

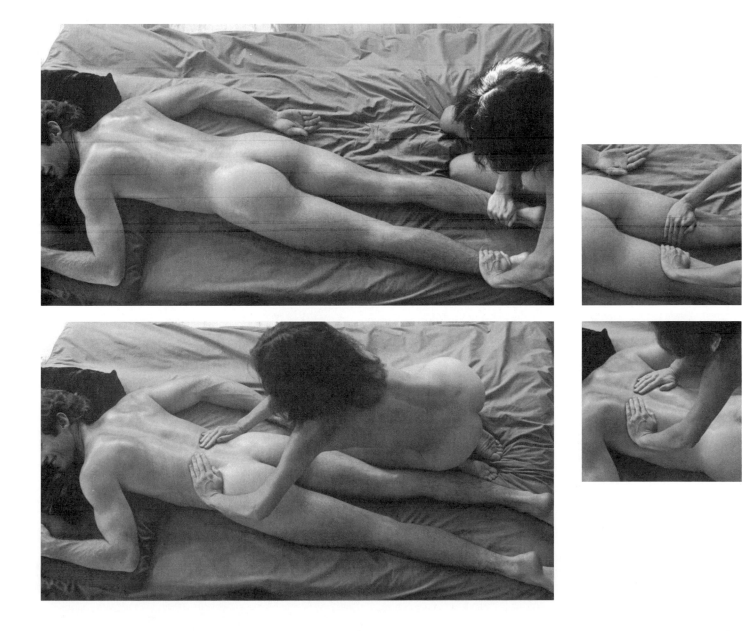

Use the whole surface of your hand throughout this stroke, making contact from your fingertips to the base of the palm. As you move straight up the legs, mold your hands to the changing shapes of your partner's legs. Reposition yourself at your partner's waist when your hands reach the buttocks. Try to do this without interrupting the stroke.

When your fingertips nearly touch at the base of the spine, the stroke merges with the back circulation movement you used at the beginning of the back massage. This time massage from your partner's side — straddling then repositioning at the feet is awkward. Move all the way up to the shoulders and return, pressing the sides of the body. At the hips simply continue straight down the outside of the thighs until you reach the ankles. Turn your hands a final time until you return to your starting position at the back of the ankles.

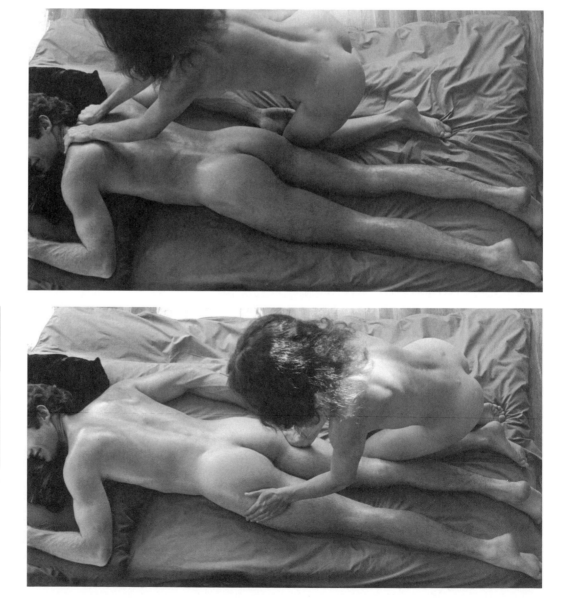

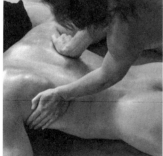

Since you're massaging large surfaces during this stroke, it's tempting to rush through the final turn on the tiny heel of the foot. But remember, your partner's foot longs to be touched. Keeping your fingers together, bend your hands to cover the sides of the foot as you turn. Attending to little details like this will make the massage unforgettable.

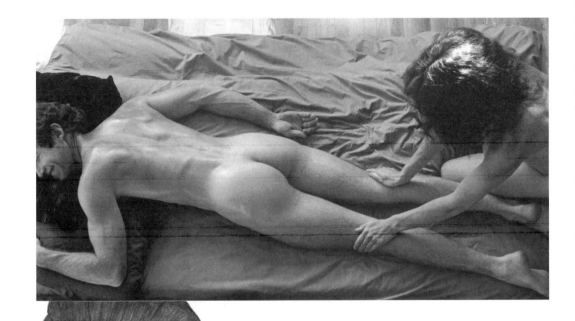

Tibial nerve

Sciatic nerve

CHAPTER 5

The Back of the Legs

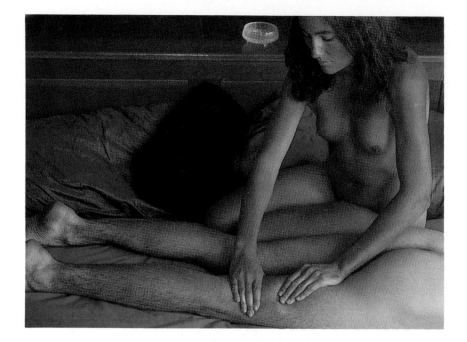

Resist the temptation to see the legs and back as completely separate entities lest you skip over crucial muscles and tendons that are shared by both. It makes sense to massage the back before the legs, because for the most part, the legs are operated from the midhip and lower back by remote control. In fact, virtually every localized movement in the body begins on an adjacent structure. Nearly all movement of the leg depends on thigh and hip girdle muscle action. The thigh itself is moved by muscles that originate on the lower part of the spine, while the gluteus maximus, the large muscle that dominates the buttocks, emerges from the bony iliac crest at the base of the spine.

Anxious to move along, masseurs often get sloppy in the gray zone between major body parts. To do so is to commit two classic errors: First, massage should never be rushed; second, the body doesn't operate in "sections," but rather as a single living organism.

Just as the leg depends on the lower back, the foot moves by remote control from the lower leg. Here the relationship with the Achilles tendon, the body's largest tendon, which descends from mid-calf muscles to wrap around the heel, is more obvious. Virtually everything that happens on the foot involves this massive tendon. Work on it now and your foot massage, the next part of the full-body massage after the back of the legs, will be far more effective.

After you've completed all of the strokes on one leg, move to the other. Your partner's entire attention is focused on your hands and the feelings they create during massage. If you break contact, she will feel abandoned. When you're interrupted or must change position, touch your partner's body. A single hand will do.

Fast Stroking the Back of the Legs

Fast stroking is part two of the luxurious tactile event that began with the full-body circulation stroke at the end of your back massage. Use this stroke to show your partner that the same kind of delicious sensation he's been experiencing on the back is moving, with great authority, to the back of the legs. In the language of touch, your hands make the points and your partner acknowledges them silently.

Move onto the limbs one at a time. Starting on the midback and descending slowly to the bottom of the feet, pull down rhythmically with one hand after the other. Keep one hand up while the other is down. Begin with generous strokes, covering half the back and nearly an entire leg with each hand. Bring your hands closer to each other and focus on a smaller area as you move down the legs. Maintain the same rhythm on the large and small strokes and your partner will feel cascading waves of sensation moving off the back onto the legs. Repeat the movement ten times. Fast stroking takes you to the ankles where you will reverse direction and begin pressing blood from an extremity to the heart.

The first stroke on the back of the legs becomes the last stroke on the back.

◆ Your hands are perfectly shaped to follow descending nerve paths while fast stroking down the sides of the body. During this full-body stroke you may want to stop for a moment. It's fine to rest during massage but be sure not to break contact with your partner. Make it a planned break, a part of the massage instead of an interruption. The rich concentra-

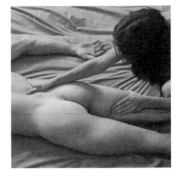

tion of nerves at the base of the spine offer an inviting place to rest your hands, one over the other. While you rest, press lightly over the lower back with the full surface of your fingers and palm. Be still. Your partner will focus all of her attention on a penetrating sensation that spreads slowly from the base of the spine. It feels warm, protective, as if your hands were meant to be there.

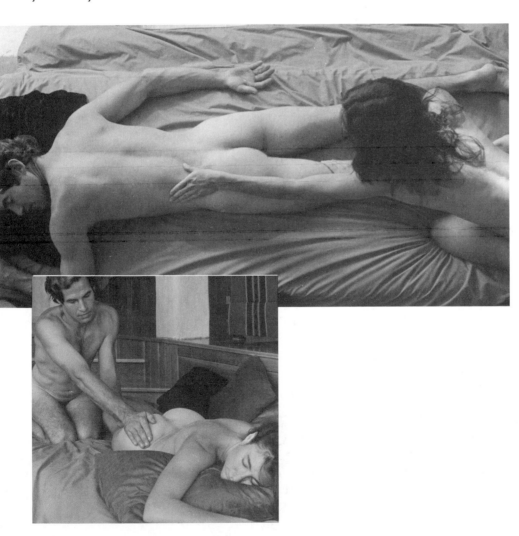

Full-Hand Stroking

One of the basic truths in massage, that a sense of well-being is closely tied to good blood circulation, makes this stroke a great favorite. If you have time for nothing else, a few minutes spent full-hand stroking each leg will leave your partner feeling energized and optimistic.

Oil the legs, buttocks, and feet before you start. Begin at the ankle with your hands cupped over the muscular portion of the calf. Keep your left hand on top on her right leg , your right hand on her left. Even when massaging thin legs be sure to maintain contact from your fingertips to the base of your palm throughout the stroke. At the ankle your fingertips may brush the massage surface; higher up on the fleshier thigh they will flatten out.

Massage the legs one at a time. Starting at the ankle, bring your hands up your partner's leg together, pressing down as you move higher. Turn your top hand across the buttocks to the side of her hip. Your bottom hand turns just below the buttocks to fit against the inside of the thigh. Bring the hands down her leg together pressing inward lightly with your fingers. Reserve deep pressures for the first part of the stroke when you're moving blood back toward the heart. Turn your hands again at her ankles and return to the starting position. Don't rush the tiny ankle turn at the bottom of the stroke, a common error. Small body parts are as hungry for sensation as large ones. Turning across the bottom of the foot insures a completed stroke while including a new part of the body.

Ten times up and down each leg; twenty, if you're feeling generous.

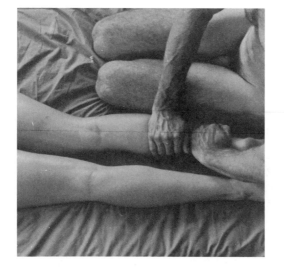
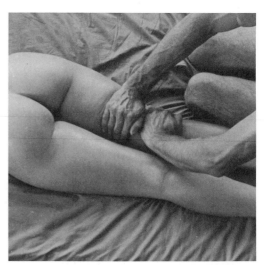

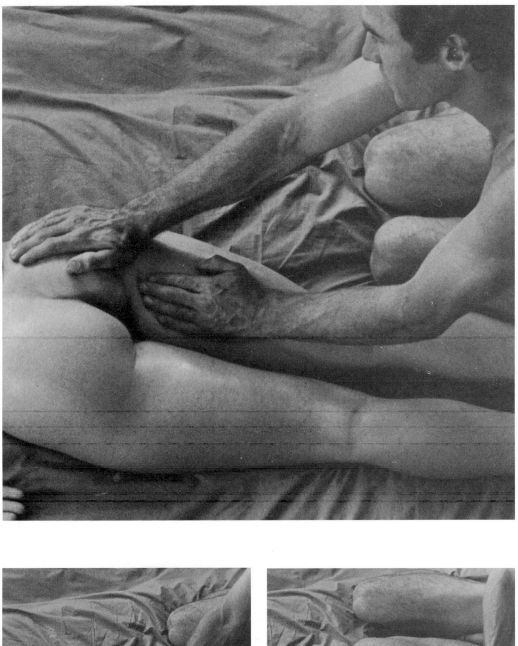

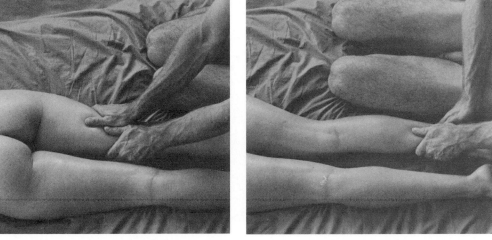

- Your partner may want small pillow support under the ankles
- Have several large soft pillows on hand for the shoulders
- Use both hands if you need to move a leg — grasp it above and below the knee
- Put your oil near your partner's knees
- On a narrow massage surface, use pillows under your own knees
- Go easy on the inside of the thigh where large blood vessels are close to the surface
- Oil the bottom of the foot when you oil the leg — your hands will brush the bottom of the foot on the long circulation strokes

Kneading the Back of the Leg

After you knead the back for awhile, the legs begin to crave the same deep penetrating feeling. Kneading's hypnotic rhythm and great adaptability makes it a great favorite everywhere on the body. If he has anything at all to say during massage, your partner learns to ask for kneading again and again. This classic full-hand stroke spreads a warm, penetrating sensation from one end of the leg to the other.

Knead the back of the leg the same way you kneaded the back — by reaching across your partner (as shown in Chapter 4). Start at the ankles and move up to the hips. Your hands move in opposing circles, one hand picking up a fold of flesh while the other opens wide. Use your thumbs to pick up flesh. Thumb squeezing is an important part of the fluid release effect, during which oxygen and blood-soluble nutrients are pumped into the tissues, while acidic irritants are removed. Use your fingertips on the calf where tissues are firmer; the thigh and buttocks will accept the whole surface of both hands. Knead up and down the leg three times so that you finish on the thigh.

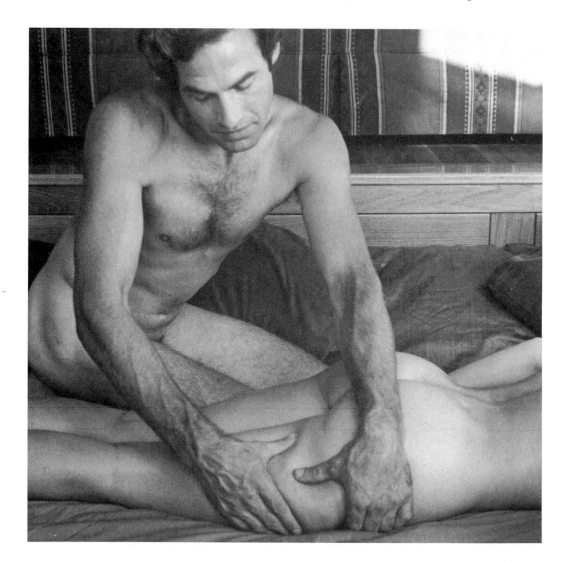

Deep Friction

If your partner has thickly muscled legs he will take special pleasure in a few minutes of deep friction. This is the stroke athletic trainers swear by. You can do it almost anywhere, with or without oil, and it travels effortlessly. Get it right and you will feel muscles deep within the leg ripple beneath your hands.

Anchor the stroke with your left hand if you're right-handed (vice versa if you're left-handed). Make a fist with your right hand and press down with the flat part of your knuckles. Remember, friction strokes never turn on the surface of the skin, only on internal tissues. Press down until you feel solid muscle tissue and rotate slowly. Move up and down the leg repositioning your hands every few inches. Go easy on the back of the knee where large blood vessels are close to the surface.

Forearm Friction

To distribute deep pressures more evenly while covering large areas like the back of the thighs, press down with your forearm. Oil the leg first — use extra oil if your partner has hairy legs. Grasp your friction arm directly over the portion that makes contact with your free arm (as shown). Press down while circling slowly. Deep friction fans always appreciate having both legs massaged at once. You can easily supply this unique feeling by simply moving your partner's legs together before you begin. Then, while moving up and down the body, make contact straight across both legs from the ankles to the hips.

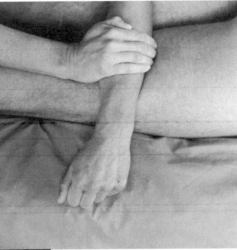

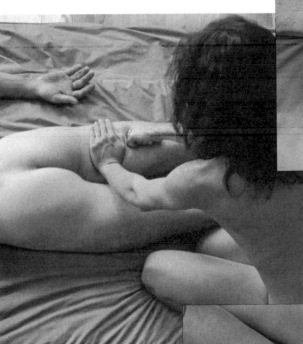

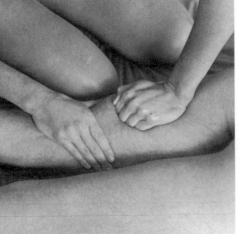

Circling the Buttocks

The large gluteus maximus muscles on the buttocks, used when climbing stairs, fold over the hamstrings on the back of the thigh. Since the gluteus maximus departs from the strictly vertical position of the hamstrings and gastrocnemius, the major leg muscles, it's massaged differently. While most strokes on the legs moved up and down, the buttocks require side-to-side or circular motions. Follow the course of the muscles with your hands.

This muscle group is better defined than most. Massage it from the base of the spine to the flattened area at the top of the hamstring muscles. Press in against the fleshy side of the buttocks with the heel of your hand to apply friction to the distinct depression at the hip joint. Turn your hand slowly.

The buttocks are a great favorite among masseurs because you can stroke deeply without disturbing internal organs or blood vessels. Use this simple friction stroke to begin massaging them.

Press down evenly so the full flat surface of your hands grips your partner's skin. Make contact from your fingertips to the base of your palms. As you turn your hands in gentle opposing circles — one hand up while the other is down — your partner's buttocks will rotate slowly. Once you get a gentle rhythm going it's fun to build up speed until your hands are turning in rapid circles.

Reach over to the hip joints and circle moderately fast, pressing down with your fingertips. Friction is the fastest way to reach deep within the body and make things happen. At the hip it stimulates the production of synovial fluid, which lubricates the interior surfaces of this massive joint.

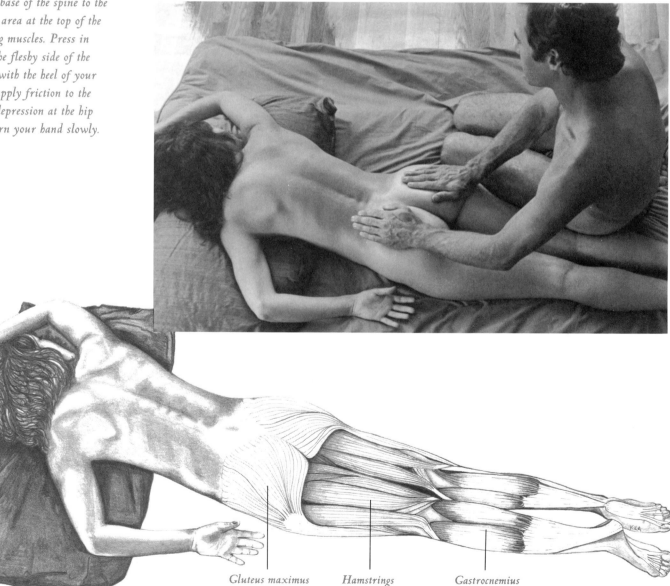

Gluteus maximus   Hamstrings   Gastrocnemius

Kneading the Buttocks

The buttocks offer an excellent opportunity to perfect your kneading technique early in the massage. Here, more than any other spot on the body, you're free of tiny structures and bony surfaces; you can knead the buttocks with the full surface of each hand.

Pick up a fold of flesh and squeeze it between your four fingers and thumb. Knead the same spot with both hands, lifting a fold of flesh with one hand as you release it with the other. Turn your hands in full circles as you knead. Move slowly from the thigh to the base of the spine up and down each side of the buttocks.

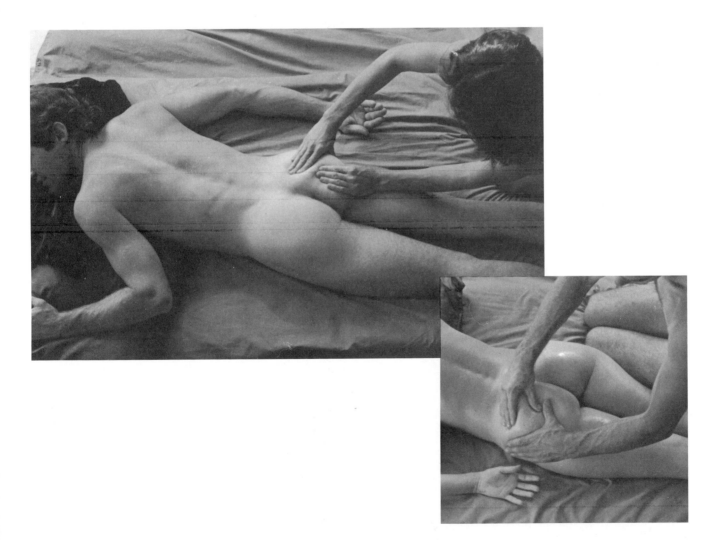

- ◆ Break every stroke at the wrist
- ◆ Get feedback on pressure and speed
- ◆ Find a comfortable rhythm and stay with it
- ◆ Add pillows (if necessary) to soften the massage surface
- ◆ Focus on muscular tissues
- ◆ Move slowly up and down the legs
- ◆ Remember: consistent rhythm matters more than speed

DON'T

- ◆ Rush, especially at the outset; slow downs are disappointing
- ◆ Strike bony structures and surface blood vessels
- ◆ Wander aimlessly or skip around
- ◆ Lean on your partner — use extra pillows, if necessary
- ◆ Explain the strokes
- ◆ Encourage conversation
- ◆ Let your hands drift apart

Knuckle Snapping

Like all percussion strokes, knuckle snapping depends on a simple cushioning effect to work properly. Never bring down the whole forearm lest your massage begin to feel more like punishment than pleasure. Bending each percussion hand at the wrist just before you make contact absorbs the force of the stroke. Your partner feels a light exhilarating tapping that travels up and down the leg.

Begin on the back of the ankle and move slowly up to the hip and back. Keep your hands close together — your thumbs should brush each other as you move up and down the leg.

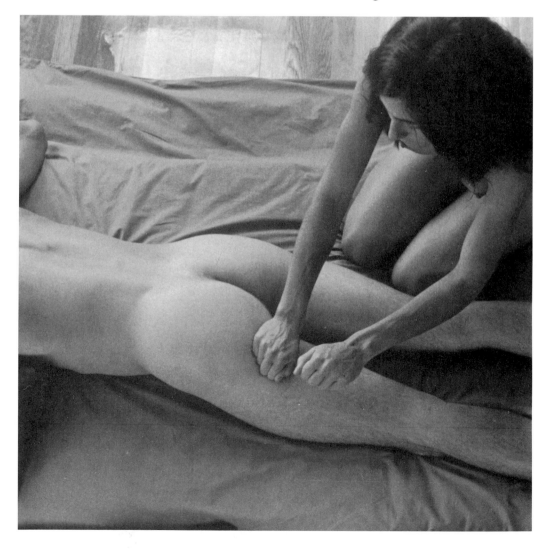

Clapping

It's easiest to massage the sides of the legs from the opposite side of the body. If you don't mind bending a bit, you can do percussion on both legs from a single side of the body. However, most masseurs prefer to reach across to the opposite leg (as shown). This full-hand percussion stroke spreads deep sensation evenly from one end of the leg to the other. Use it to energize a lethargic limb. Each stroke breaking at the wrist, your hands create a tiny vacuum as they clap. When you hear a popping sound on impact, you've got the stroke right. Move up and down the top of the leg, then reach forward and do the sides.

Thumping

People crave thumping as long as you direct the strokes carefully. Like all percussion strokes, thumping is intelligent vibration. Focus on muscular tissues but avoid bony structures and surface blood vessels. And don't stop with a single stroke. The various percussion movements complement each other so naturally that your partner will hardly notice the difference between, say, a minute of clapping and a short pounding sequence.

This stroke is identical to the thumping movement you used on the lower back (see page 47). Follow the path that you used for clapping up and down the leg. Pound out a light pattern on the top of the leg, then reach across and vibrate the far side of the opposite leg.

For a more penetrating pounding effect, strike even harder against the back of your hand (as shown). Your fingers provide double cushioning: The extra force is absorbed by both your wrist and fingers.

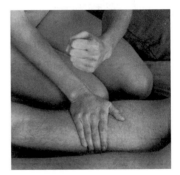

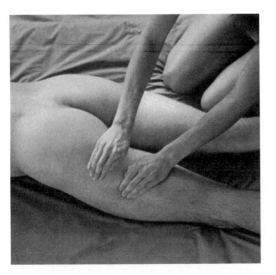

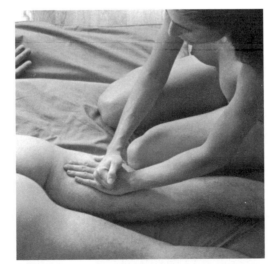

Flexing the Legs

Leg lifts give you a way to move massage from one leg to another with great drama. First your partner feels his lower legs float through the air. Tiny ligaments deep within the knees get relief. Then both legs leave the ground and the entire lower half of the body executes an exuberant backward bend at the hip.

First, flex the legs one at a time. Anchor the stroke at the back of your partner's knee with your free hand and grasp the leg at the ankle (as shown). Press just to the point where you feel muscles and tendons tighten — the point of tension — and release slowly. Pressing the bottom half of the leg forward flexes tiny ligaments within the body's most complex joint, the knee. As you repeat the stroke four or five times, you may feel the point of tension recede slightly as the ligaments and tendons are stretched gently.

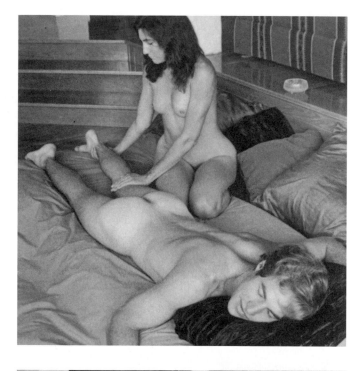

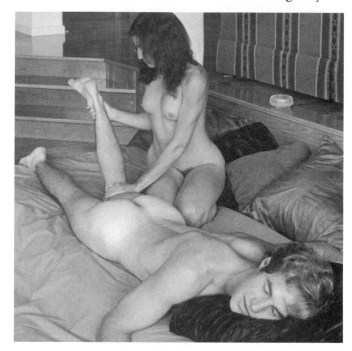

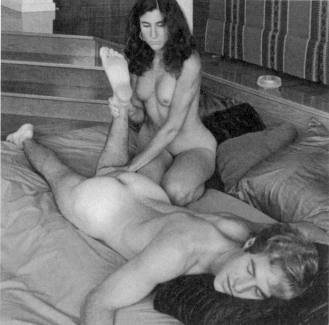

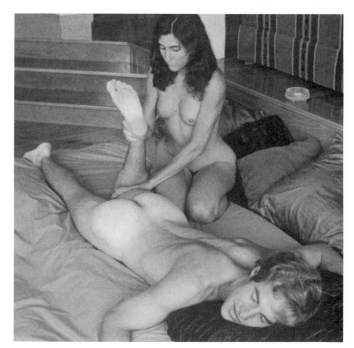

To flex both legs at once, grasp both of your partner's legs at the ankles, lift slowly and press forward with your forearm. Anchor the legs with your free hand to keep them together. Press forward slowly to the point of tension, then lower the legs to the massage surface.

Passive exercises incorporate simple antigravity effects — your partner should feel as though her leg is floating through the air effortlessly. Generally, when you move a limb it's best to provide support on both sides of the central joint. During this stroke, however, you need only support the lower leg, since your partner's knee rests firmly on the ground. Use both hands to lower the legs to the fully extended starting position. You've made your point; the other leg has now experienced massage and is ready and waiting for what comes next. However, if you're feeling muscular, try leg rotation (one of the few massage strokes where strength matters) before you begin.

JOINT FLEXING

♦ You will flex joints on every part of the body. Ask your partner for feedback on pressure and speed. Get it right now and you won't have to ask again later in the massage.

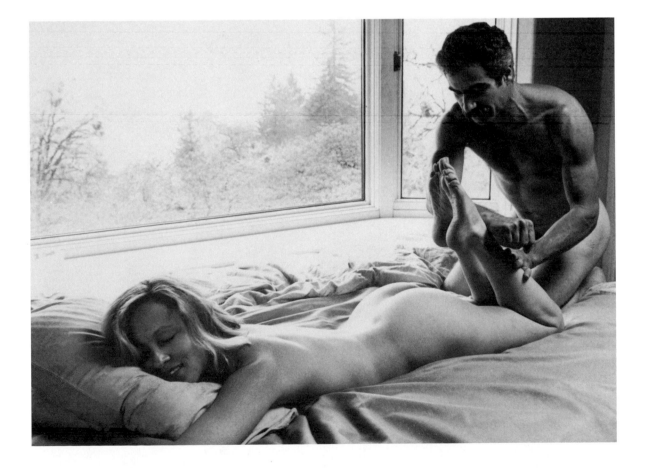

The Back of the Legs **65**

Rotating the Legs

Supporting both sides of the knee effectively "locks" your partner's legs into a single lever. You can then rotate the entire lower half of her body in backward circles from the hip joint. This stroke creates sensations that cannot be experienced outside of massage; your partner is entering new sensual territory. Let her savor the feeling.

Hold her legs above and below the knees and bring both of them straight up (as shown) — her whole lower body will follow. Here again, you will feel a point of tension as you turn. Work within it. Make three moderately large circles in each direction before returning her legs to the massage surface and repeating the strokes in this chapter on the other leg.

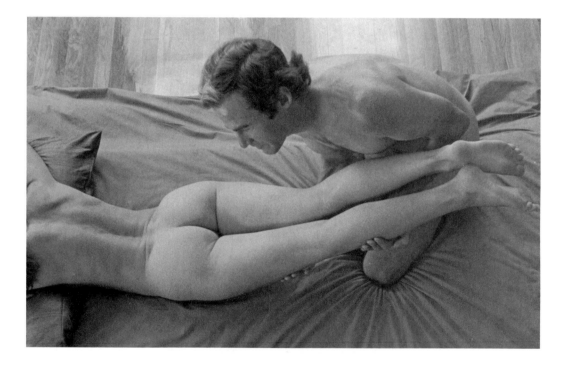

The Hip Roll

By stabilizing your partner's leg above and below the knee, her whole leg becomes a natural handle, a lever with which you can flex the massive hip joint at the top of the leg.

Support your partner's upper body at the bottom of the spine by pressing gently with the flat part of your hand. Your hand should create a steadying effect, similar to the anchoring movement during friction; the upper body remains still while the hip joint turns.

Reach in from below your partner's knee and grasp the inside of her thigh. Cradle her extended knee on your forearm during the hip roll. Starting with both of your partner's knees together, lift and rotate her leg in small circles. As you turn the leg the hip joint will follow your hands. In fact, the hip's network of tendons and ligaments will control the limits of this stroke. Feel for the various points of tension and rotate just inside them. Turn the leg three times in each direction, then lower it slowly to the massage surface.

LIFTING TIPS

◆ Style matters while lifting and lowering the leg. Short, jerky motions detract from the sensual, rolling feeling; move the leg in a graceful arc. Never lean forward onto your anchor hand. Keep the stroke focused on your partner's hip. Sometimes, you can hear the bones roll.

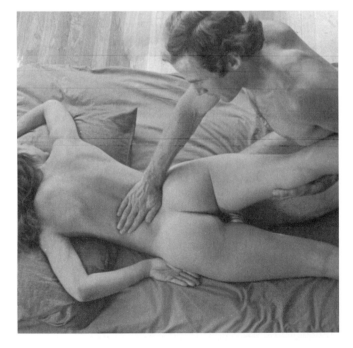

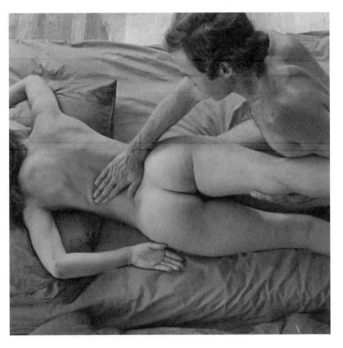

CHAPTER 6

The Feet

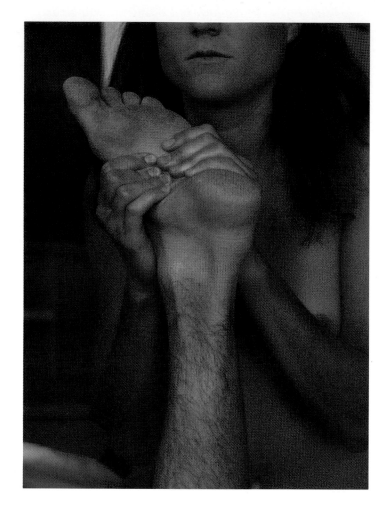

After the long strokes that swept back and forth across the back of the body, the foot is a study in detail. Using precise fingertip strokes, you will massage tiny structures here. Take your time and watch the impact that scrupulous attention to a small body part makes during massage.

If massage teaches us anything, it is that the whole body is sensually programmed. Perhaps the human body is meant to be massaged regularly. And if it's not, we lose a fundamental emotional stability that cannot be put right by exercise, pills, or therapy.

The feet have secret needs. We know that the body has been un-ambiguously programmed to respond to your life-style. The muscles, for example, are imprinted with a use 'em or lose 'em message. You don't need to break the genetic code to understand that muscles are clearly designed to be used. However, anatomical evidence suggests that we have an equally obvious message imprinted in the feet, an unmistakable recipe for pleasure. This tiny area has far more nerve endings than the back and legs combined. You saw how much your partner enjoyed massage on the back and legs, insensitive portions of the body

compared to the feet. Feet are designed to feel much more than the back and legs combined. Although the feet present a small area, be sure to take your time — every stroke counts.

Start by massaging the nerve-rich bottom of the foot, perhaps the body's most ignored area. Bound and gagged, in leather throughout the day, the bottom of the foot is usually permitted to feel little or nothing. You're about to change all that . . .

TIBIAL NERVE TAKES EXTRA PRESSURE

◆ The tibial nerve, that you first massaged on the back of the legs, bends across the arch and branches out to supply the nerve-rich sole of the foot. This area combines the body's thickest skin with the greatest number of nerve endings. Use extra pressure here — the foot can take it. Whether you're pressing down with the tips of your thumbs or the heel of your hand, your partner will welcome the feeling.

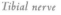

Tibial nerve

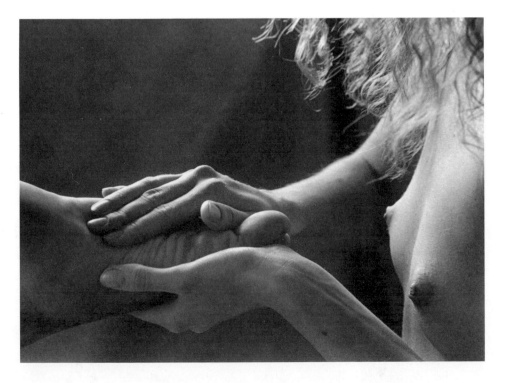

Rotating the Top of the Foot

The complex joint at the middle of the foot does not rotate in a perfect circle. Feel the joint before you rotate it. Kneel at your partner's feet. Lift one foot straight up and grasp it firmly at the ankle. Fold your free hand over the toes and wiggle the top half of the foot. Gently turn the top of the foot completely around one time in order to feel the various points of resistance that create a kind of irregular arc as you turn. Then, following the arc, rotate the top of the foot three times in each direction just inside the point of tension. As you rotate, pull outward to the point of tension. Wiggle, turn, rotate, and pull.

Knuckle Pressing the Arch

Sore feet usually mean sore arches, simply because the arch bears more weight than any other part of the body. This stroke reverses the great pressures that are focused on a few small bones and muscles all through the day. It brings unexpected relief and the realization of just how much the arches crave reverse pressure. If any stroke will encourage feedback, this one will. Listen carefully the moment you stop. Mixed with moans of pleasure you may hear the word "more."

Kneel along side of your partner and fold the leg back (as shown). Hold the top of the foot with one hand while you press down into the arch with the flat part of your knuckles. Make small circles at the deepest part of the arch. Press down firmly, the arch is built to take plenty of pressure.

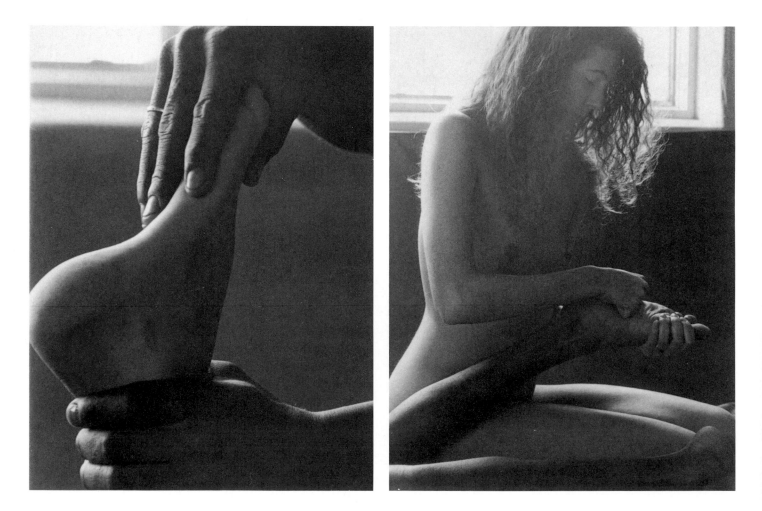

Thumb Kneading the Bottom of the Foot

Continue massaging the bottom of the foot from the same elevated position you used for knuckle pressing.

The arch is too narrow to knead with the whole hand and too firm for the fingertips. Once again, however, your body is perfectly suited for massaging this unusual surface. Your thumbs, the strongest part of your hands, fit perfectly into the hollow of the arch. Thumb kneading allows you to concentrate pressures on a small area, ideal for the bottom of the foot. Knead from both sides of the foot to reach the whole surface of the arch, the heel, and the ball of the foot with your thumbs.

Have your partner turn over during thumb kneading. That way, you can continue with the same stroke when you begin massaging the top of the foot.

Grasp the top of your partner's foot with all four fingers of each hand and press down into the center of the arch with your thumbs. Keep the thumbs as close as possible to each other. Circle with the thumbs together. If you're forced to separate them on the wider parts of the foot, keep the tips close. The thumbs should circle together while making alternative up-and-down motions. As you circle, one thumb tip should be up while the other is down.

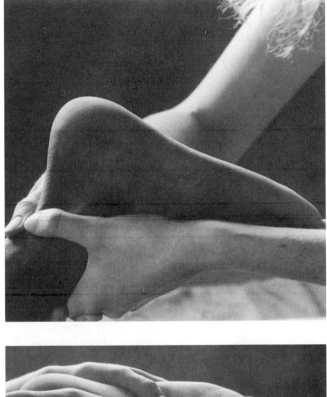

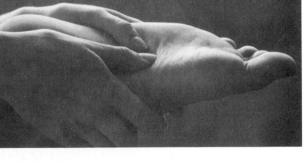

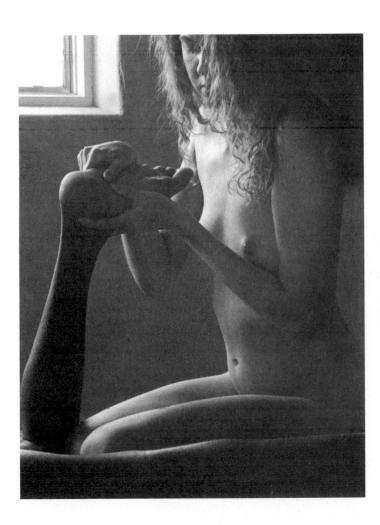

◆ Without engaging in conversation or opening her eyes, your partner should turn over midway through the foot massage. A whispered phrase, or better yet, a pleasing sound or musical tone, will signal her that the time has come to massage the front of the body. Be sure to maintain contact with your partner while she turns over. You will begin to massage on the front of the body, starting on the top of the feet and ending, about forty minutes later, on the head.

Circulation

If sore feet means massaging the arches, a sluggish mood should bring the other side of the foot to your attention. The blood reaches its furthest point from the heart at the feet, where it tends to pool during periods of inactivity. Nothing picks up the spirits like a few minutes of steady foot circulation.

The blood supply to the foot emerges from the lower leg via two large arteries. The top one stretches visibly across the center of the foot bending over to the big toe. The other crosses the outside bottom edge of the foot to the little toe. Blood is returned to the heart in the roughly parallel venous system. This stroke stimulates both systems at once, oxygenating the tissues of the foot and clearing acidic wastes that cause fatigue.

Foot circulation works the same way as the larger circulation movements on the back of the leg. Although your hands move only a few inches here, be sure to place them so the top hand can turn across the ankle. Kneel or sit at your partner's feet. Cup your hands over the top of one foot, keeping your right hand on top on the left foot, vice versa on the other foot. Make sure to wrap your fingers around the side of the foot. Press up first with one hand and then the other, turning at the ankle and returning along the side of the foot to your starting position.

It's fun to vary the movement by delivering thirty fast hand-over-hand strokes up to the ankle. This time skip the return part of the circulation stroke on the side of the foot. Concentrate on pressing blood up toward the heart. Build up speed for a final dozen high-speed circulation strokes, bringing your foot massage to a sensual exclamation point.

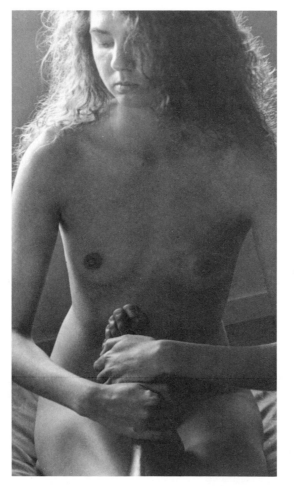

Friction

The foot is supplied with a number of convenient natural handles that make massage easier. Hold the heel with one hand while applying friction with the other. Keep the foot steady while you apply friction with your fingertips (as shown). Pressing lightly, move around the ankle making tiny circles, first in one direction then the other. Press down harder around the heel where thick tissues will accept deeper pressure.

◆ You cannot imagine what a profound difference a good foot massage can make to your mood, until you experience it yourself. Stress has little power over a man or woman with completely relaxed feet.

Be sure to include the feet when you massage any part of the body, particularly if your partner has been tense. Afterward, most people will have trouble remembering what it was they were worried about before you started and where it used to hurt.

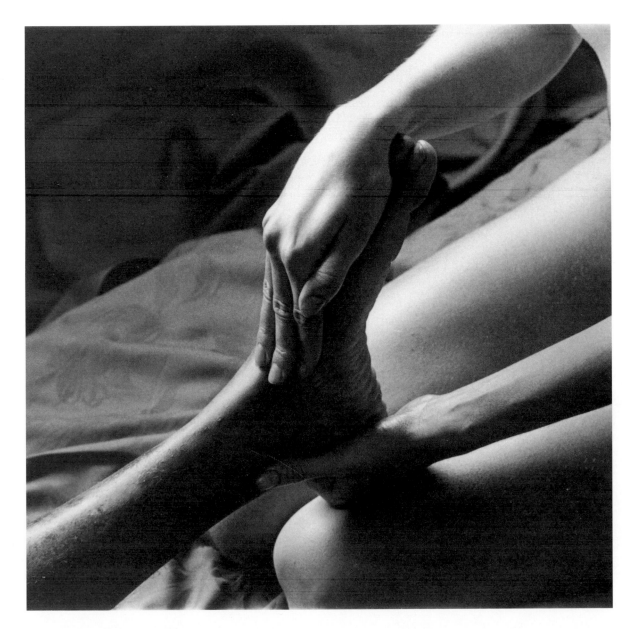

Toes

The notion that only big body parts are worthy of massage is old and false. Skip the toes and the toes will notice.

In fact, the toes should be massaged individually. Toe massage can serve as an interesting prelude to the fingers, because you do things in both places that simply aren't possible anywhere else on the body. The best strokes focus on the remarkably sensitive sides of the toes. You may want to support each foot with a small pillow behind the ankle before you begin. Don't rush — repeat movements three times, once to get the toes used to being touched, twice more so they enjoy it.

Pull down the sides of each toe in a corkscrew motion, twisting your fingers in a half circle from the bottom of the toe to the top. Then pull straight up the sides. Grasp the end of the toe and rotate it in both directions. Finally, fold your hand over the end of the toes (as shown) and flex them gently forward and back, just inside the point of tension.

Toe massage sends your partner an important message: You care enough to massage the toes individually.

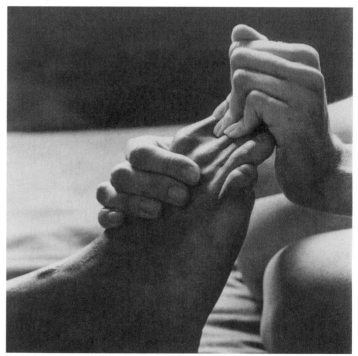

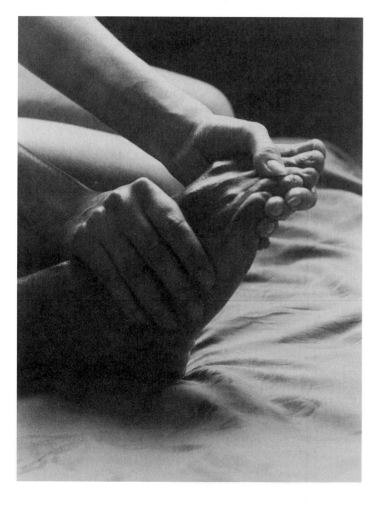

Ankle Friction

Now that you've massaged the foot with circulation and kneading movements, you've completed the first part of a fluid release sequence. Complete it by going directly to the lymph nodes that drain the foot on the inside of the ankle. Remember, the lymph system has no heart to help circulate fluids. Massage drains toxins from the body that might otherwise take weeks to be expelled.

Lifting the foot at the heel puts tension on the large Achilles tendon, which runs up the back of the calf. But raising the tiny arch just *above* the heel lets your partner's foot fall back to a relaxed position while his leg rises. Wrap all four of your fingers around the arch (as shown) and bring it up slowly. The foot feels relaxed and supple when you lift it with this natural handle. Elevate the foot with one hand while applying friction around the ankle with the other.

Brush your partner's feet with your fingertips, breaking contact for a moment on the tips of the toes. Reach forward and grasp the leg, midcalf. Maintaining contact, pause for a moment while your partner's sensate focus moves from the foot to the leg.

HISTORICAL MASSAGE

"In Europe, massage is found everywhere, and many 'wise men' (or women) in the country or in towns have it to thank for their best 'miraculous cures.'"

Emil A.G. Kleen, M.D., *Massage and Medical Gymnastics* (London: J.A. Churchill, 1918), p. 13.

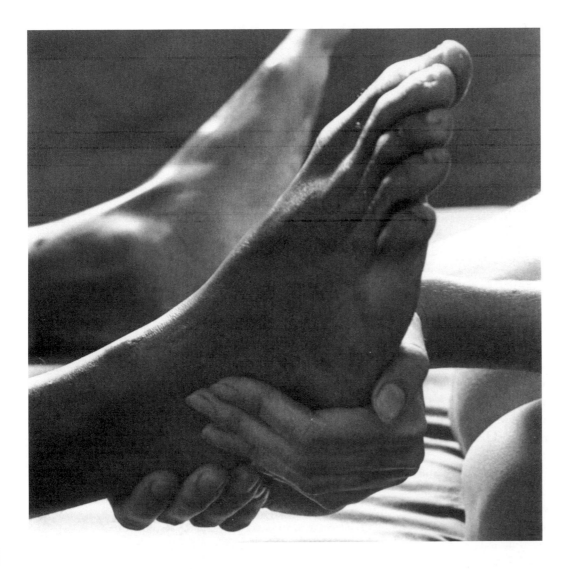

CHAPTER 7

The Front of the Legs

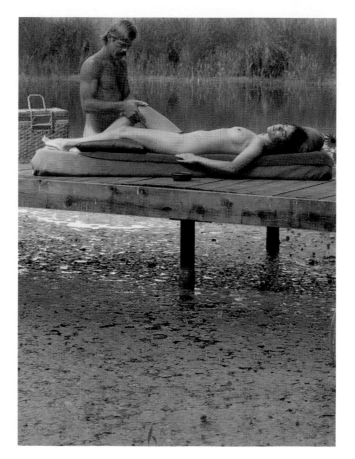

*I*f your partner is fatigued, stressed, or simply sedentary, blood tends to pool in the legs . . . thereby generating more stress and fatigue. You are what you feel; to improve a bad mood or vanquish fatigue, massage the legs. This part of the full-body massage completes the process you began on the back of the legs: creating a massive fluid release effect from the feet to the hips. Acidic wastes and toxins are cleared from internal tissues while the blood supply of the legs is super-oxygenated. Your partner will feel the difference in minutes. The legs, suddenly animated, seem weightless. The whole body is infused with renewed energy and zest. You must experience these strokes to believe how effective fluid release leg massage can be in transforming a sluggish body and calming a stressed one. And you will soon enough — your reward for giving this full-body massage cannot be far off.

You can do two special things for your partner on the front of the legs: First, by oxygenating the internal tissues, you turn negative feelings into sunny optimism; second, you can concentrate a variety of friction and fingertip kneading strokes on the knee, the body's most complex joint. More on that soon.

Circulation

From your starting point at the ankles, the front of the legs point straight ahead to the heart. You now have the best opportunity yet to influence one of the body's basic mechanisms: blood circulation. By pressing blood up through the large veins of the legs without speeding up the heart, you can alter the fundamental pace of your partner's body. Again, this stroke maps out new sensual territory; the sensation of blood warming the legs without help from the circulatory system cannot be experienced outside of massage.

Cup both your hands over one ankle while wrapping your fingers around the sides of the leg (as shown). Be sure to make contact with your fingertips. As you move toward the heart, press your index fingers and thumbs tightly enough to push a fold of flesh before them. Spread your thumbs to accommodate the fleshy portion of the thigh.

Turn at the top of the thigh — bring the inner hand around the top of the leg while the outer one moves up higher across the hip itself. Bring your outside hand down so the fingertips are parallel with the inside hand. Then pull down the legs with both hands using light pressure. Use firm pressure going up the legs, but make superficial contact with light pressure going down. Turn both hands a final time at the ankle and reposition them for the beginning of the stroke. Don't rush the turn. Make contact with as much of your hand as possible across the ankles and onto the top of the leg.

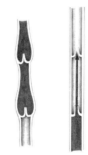

Tiny one-way valves in the capillaries allow blood to return to the heart without back-flowing. When circulation is sluggish, blood pools above the valves, visibly distending the capillary walls.

Circulation strokes force open the valves and tone the capillaries while slowing down the heart, an effect that cannot be duplicated outside massage.

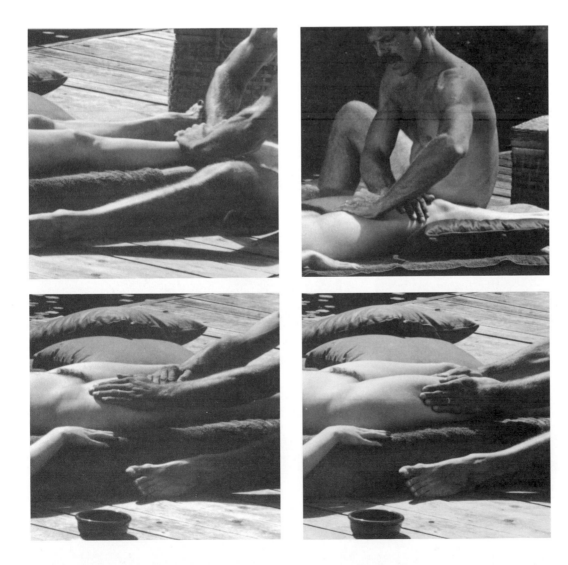

The Calf Twist

Oil your forearm before you begin this stroke. Raise your partner's leg (as shown) to completely relax the calf muscles. Anchor the stroke at her ankle by grasping it with your free hand. Reaching around the calf, clench your fist and rotate the fleshy inside of your forearm on the relaxed muscle. Move up and down the calf, rotating in slow circles from the back of the ankles to the back of the knee.

Forearm meets calf — when was the last time that happened?

The Thigh Twist

Keep your partner's knee raised for another course of forearm twisting. The stroke you used on the calf travels naturally to the thigh, where muscles are thicker. By massaging the thigh with a similar stroke, you can extend the same agreeable sensation from the bottom of the leg to the top. Again, anchor the stroke at the ankle while reaching forward with your free arm. Rotate your forearm on the thick thigh muscles, circling slowly as you move up and down from the knee to the hip.

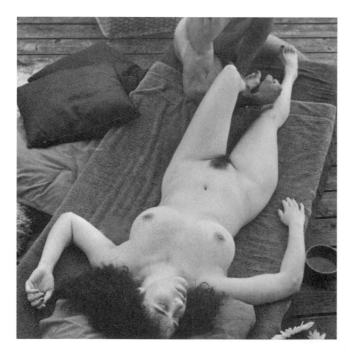 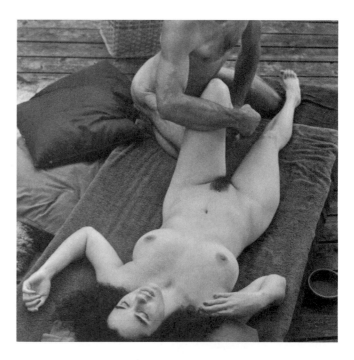

Kneading the Calf

With the leg raised, the calf can be kneaded in ways that were impossible on the back of the leg. Don't be afraid of confusing your partner. Kneading the back of the leg from the front adds intelligence and wit to your full-body massage. Do it now because you can.

This unusual thumb-kneading stroke works on both sides of the leg at once to reach the sides of the large muscle you just circled with your forearm. You will use it again at the knee to massage tiny ligaments that tie the top and bottom of the leg together.

Grasp the calf muscles with all four fingers of each hand and knead along the upper edge with your thumbs (as shown). Unlike most kneading strokes, your thumbs will not brush each other here. Nevertheless, make symmetrical circles with each thumb on opposite sides of the leg. While you knead, imagine that the thumbs can touch and your hands will synchronize — one thumb up while the other is down — easily.

SENSATION ENHANCERS

- Oil the whole leg before massaging any part of it
- Add extra oil if your partner has hairy legs
- Spend extra time on the knee, the body's most complex joint
- Knead the sides of the leg right down to the massage surface
- Use light pressure on the inside of the thigh where the femoral artery is close to the surface
- Grip the leg above and below the knee whenever you raise and lower it

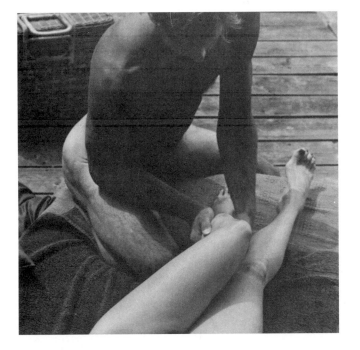

Rotating the Front of the Legs

Thanks to the locking joints at the knees, half the body will rise when you pick up the legs at the ankles. Anything that rises that easily fairly cries out to be rotated.

Indeed, the legs are made for this massage stroke — you will find another natural handle below the calf muscle, directly behind the ankles, that fits your hand per- fectly. Lift there with one hand and on the lower part of the calf muscle with the other. Pick up both legs at once, then rotate them in a slow circle up to your shoulders and down to your waist.

Two of the leg's three major joints remain rigid during this stroke. The body's largest bones are locked in place at the knee while the ankle rests against your hand. Lift and turn the leg just above the ankle and the hip joint will rotate with your hands (see illustration below).

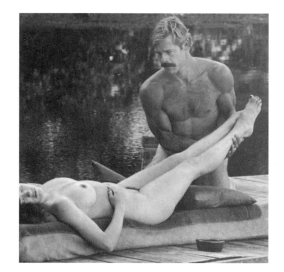

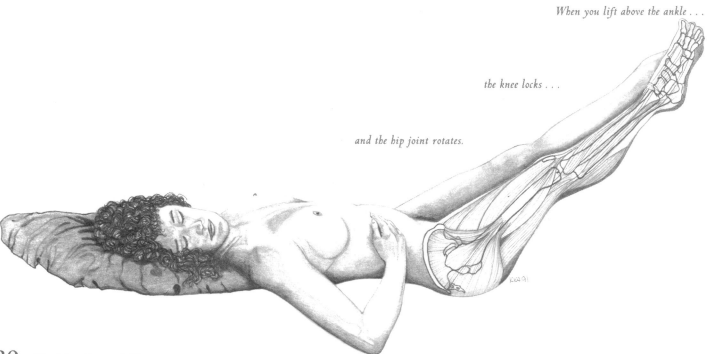

When you lift above the ankle . . .

the knee locks . . .

and the hip joint rotates.

Flexing the Knees

Begin knee massage by flexing the leg at the knee and hip while gently stretching the massive four-part quadriceps on the front of the thigh.

Lift one of your partner's legs at the ankle. As it rises, press forward slowly with your forearm on the front of the knee. When you feel resistance — the point of tension — reverse the stroke, unfolding the leg until it lies flat before you. Repeat the pressing cycle three times, moving your partner's leg through the folding and unfolding motions smoothly, as though she were swimming. Avoid sudden jerky motions.

Near the top of the stroke you may feel the point of tension recede slightly as muscles and tendons are stretched gently.

Lift and press each leg individually, then lift both legs by reaching behind the ankles (as shown) and press forward on the front of the knees. Again, return the legs to the full flat position each time you press forward on the knees. Repeat three times.

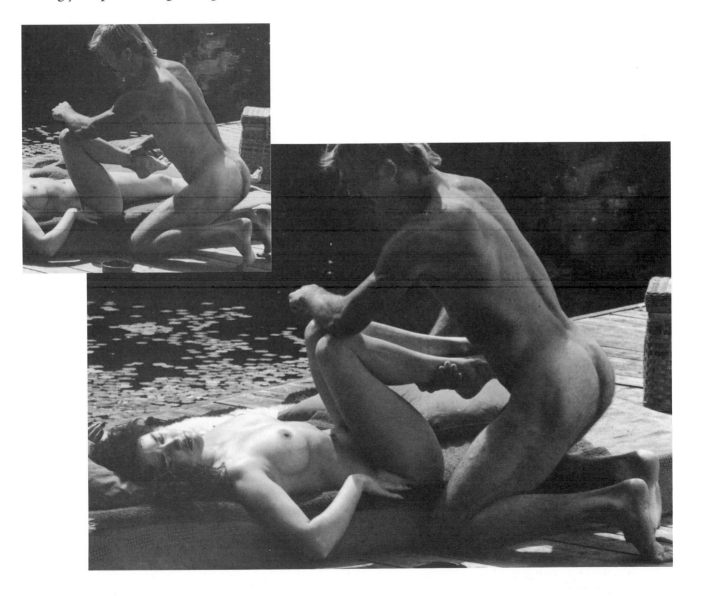

Resist the temptation to treat the knee as a mere bony impediment. Yes, the thigh, with its fleshy expanse and well-defined muscles, lies just ahead. Nevertheless, you will do your partner a great disservice if you skip over the knee, as some masseurs do.

Fingertip Kneading the Knee

Rising from the front of the leg like the head of a mushroom, the kneecap seems to float above the powerful muscles of the leg. Knead around the bony edge, pressing inward slightly with the tips of your thumbs.

Fold your fingers around the bottom of the leg and reach forward with your thumbs (as shown) while rotating them in opposing circles. Begin just below the kneecap, separating your thumbs as you move up the sides of the knee. Feel the texture of the kneecap with the side of your thumbs as you knead, but avoid pressing directly on the kneecap. Move forward slowly, covering each side of the knee thoroughly.

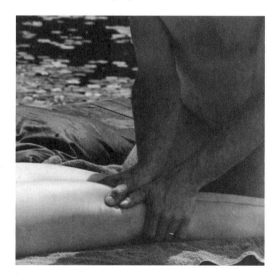

Your thumbs will meet again at the top of the kneecap where the massive four-part quadriceps end. Give that spot extra attention before separating your thumbs once again and reversing the stroke. Move down the sides of the knee, kneading as you go. Your thumbs will meet again at the bottom of the kneecap, where you begin the whole stroke again. Repeat this cycle three times.

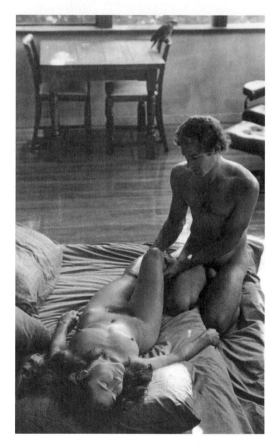

The largest bones in the body focus powerful forces on the knee from above and below.

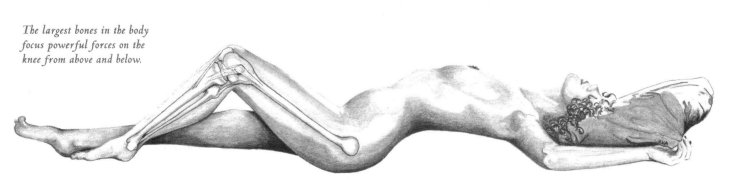

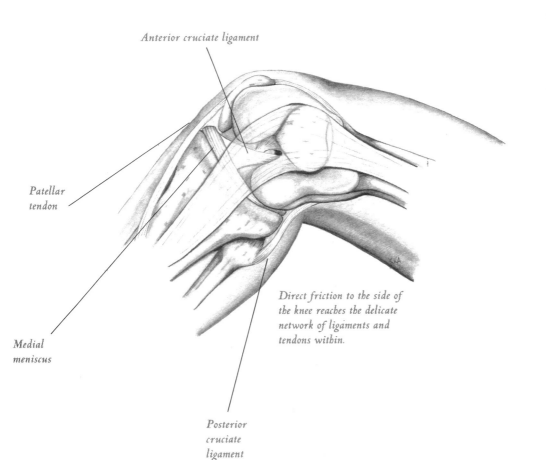

Anterior cruciate ligament

Patellar
tendon

Medial
meniscus

Direct friction to the side of
the knee reaches the delicate
network of ligaments and
tendons within.

Posterior
cruciate
ligament

Most front-of-the-leg massage
can be viewed as a preparation
for massaging the knee, the body's
most complex and vulnerable
joint. Unlike the hip and arm
joints, which are joined on one
side to the trunk, the knee stands
alone. With the body's largest
bones precariously hinged here,
powerful forces are focused on
this spot from above and below.
The joint is meant to move forward and back while permitting
a slight lateral motion in both
directions. Push it too hard and
rubber band–like structures
within give way. Even under
ideal conditions the leg's largest
muscles tug on tiny internal ligaments and tendons within the
knee. The more you can relax
the muscles of the leg first, the
better your chance of relaxing
the knee itself.

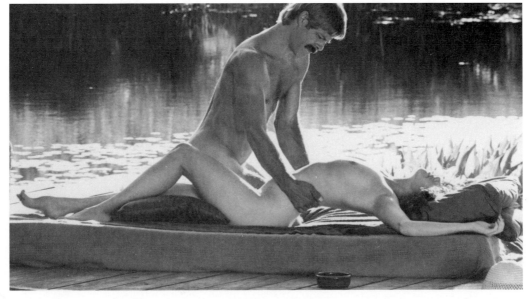

Fast Stroking the Knee

While traveling up and down the side of the knee, this simple friction stroke transmits warm sensations deep within.

Raise your partner's legs to bring the knees straight up before you (as shown). Keeping your fingers together, press your hands against the sides of the knee. Start well below the kneecap and move both hands up until your thumbs are parallel with the top of the knee. Move back and forth in a fast full-hand friction stroke.

Knuckle Pressing the Top of the Knee

Most places on the body where large structures intersect with very small ones are buried beneath the ribs or skull, completely outside the reach of massage. However, the spot where the quadriceps meet the knee rises to meet your hands as you move up the leg. Use this stroke to focus on the knot of muscle on top of the knee until you feel a tangible easing of tension. Get into an easy rhythm that you can maintain for several minutes, if necessary.

Anchor your partner's leg behind the knee with one hand and apply friction with the other. Make a fist and rotate the flat part of your knuckle against the knobby muscular bump just above the knee. Rotate three times first in one direction, then the other.

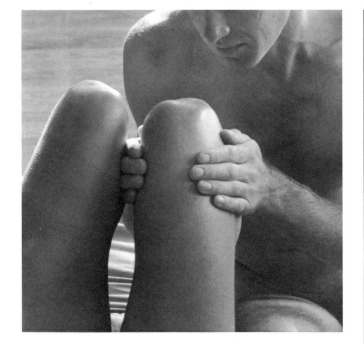

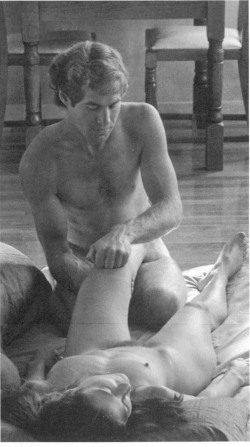

Circling the Knee

Begin in the same position you used for fingertip kneading — fingers wrapped around the knee and pointed down, thumbs tucked under the kneecap — but this time circle the kneecap with your thumbs. Starting on opposite sides of the knee, pull straight back until your thumbs cross each other at the bottom of the kneecap. At that point each thumb crosses onto the other side of the knee, where it travels straight up to the top. Cross thumbs again at the top of the knee and pull down to the starting position. Circle the knee three times in each direction, pressing lightly against the kneecap throughout the stroke. Although you can move in either direction when you circle, the sequence usually works best if you pull downward with both thumbs when starting.

Use light, even pressure all the way around your partner's knee. Never "dig in" beneath the kneecap with the tips of your thumbs. At the end of the stroke, gradually release the pressure. Maintaining superficial contact, make a final circle and trace the path around the kneecap.

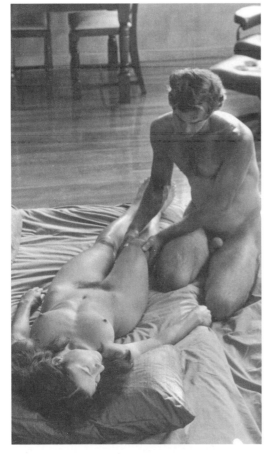

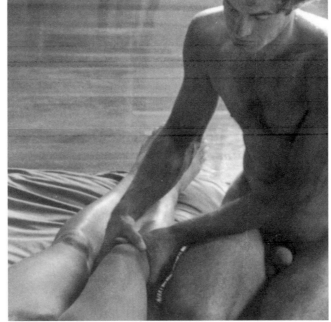

Flexing the Leg

Massage puts people together in unpredictable ways. Here on the front of the leg you have a chance to test the condition of a major nerve on the back of the leg. Once you get yourself properly wrapped around your partner, pressing forward on the top of her foot tightens muscles up and down the back of the thigh and calf. A pinched nerve will immediately make this leg-flexing uncomfortable. Normally, however, your partner won't be thinking much about the sciatic nerve during a stroke that feels as though she is standing on her toes while lying on her back. As her whole leg floats up into the air the toes curl and the muscles on the back of the leg are stretched gently. Watch for the slow smile of sensual awareness as she gets comfortable with this newest feeling.

Wrap your arm around your partner's knee and, turning your hand inward, grasp her thigh (as shown). Support her leg at the knee joint with your arm. Then, while stretching the whole leg straight out, bend the top of the foot forward to the point of tension with your free hand.

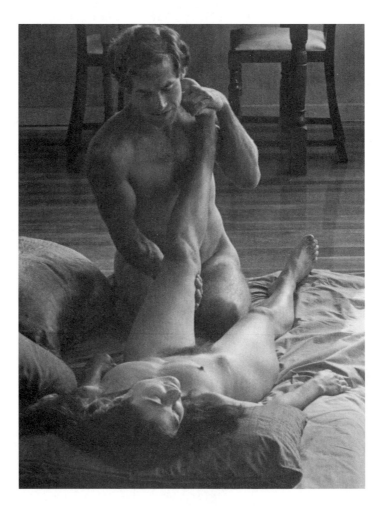

Kneading the Side of the Leg

The fleshy expanse of the thigh offers one of the best opportunities for kneading anywhere on the body. Knead the side of the leg the same way you kneaded the back of the legs and the back, by reaching over from the opposite side of your partner's body (as shown). Start at the hips with a vigorous full-hand stroke. Each time one of your hands makes a circle, pick up a generous fold of flesh with your thumb.

Move down to the knee, kneading deeply. In order to continue down the side of the calf, full-hand kneading gives way to a fingertip stroke below the knee. On the calf, your thumbs will pick up a tiny fold of flesh each time you open and close your fingers. Maintain the same rhythm with your fingertips that you used for the whole hand. Continue kneading to the ankle, then reverse your direction and move back up to the hip.

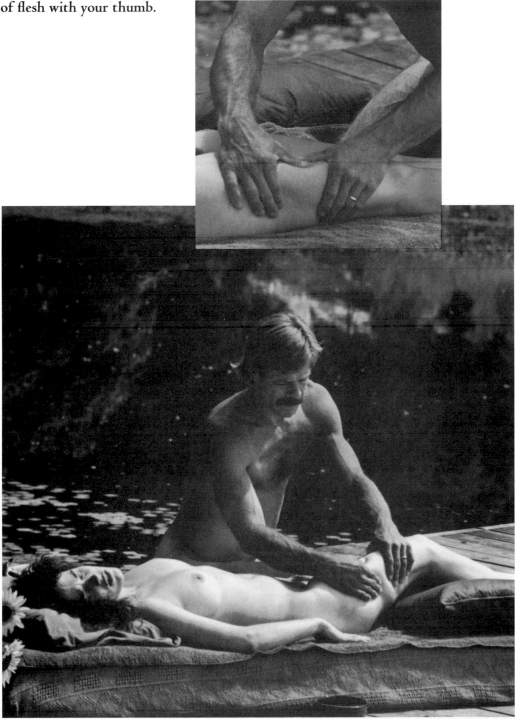

Hip Friction

The joint at the hip, the largest in the body, is buried beneath a webbing of powerful muscles and tendons. Unlike the joints at the wrist, knee, and elbow, you cannot easily touch it. Most massage movements glide over or around the hip joint; this full-hand friction movement presses right in to the center of the joint.

Relax the structures that are attached to the joint before you massage the hip itself. Start below the hip with a full-hand friction stroke to the flat muscles on the side of the leg. Pressing down moderately hard, make small circles with your fingers. Move up slowly until you feel the knobby top of the femur, the leg's largest bone. The hip joint is just above that point and slightly inward, toward the spine. You may not be able to precisely locate the joint, but work over the whole area with deep friction and the hip will work better when you stop. Any friction movement in the area stimulates production of synovial fluid, the important joint lubricant.

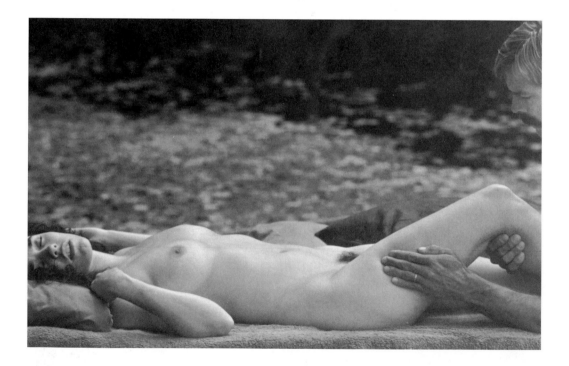

Clapping

Nothing will brighten up your partner's mood more quickly than well-oxygenated legs. No matter how many pills you gobble, feelings of depression and moodiness will remain if blood pools in the legs. The nation's psychiatry bill would be significantly lower if this simple fact were widely recognized. Awaken and refresh the legs with massage and the whole body will follow.

Clapping works best on the thick muscular outside of the thighs. Move onto the top of the legs briefly; however, stay off the top of the knee and the inside of the thigh, where a rare surface artery makes percussion inadvisable. Whether you make contact with the side or the top of the leg, the vibrations will carry right through to stimulate the tissues you cannot reach.

Reach across to the opposite side of your partner's body to do this stroke. Cup your hands slightly and bring them down one at a time in quick succession, breaking each "blow" at the wrist. Use light to moderate pressure, just enough to bring a warm glow to the skin. Keep your hands close enough for the thumbs to brush each other as you massage. Move up and down the outside of the thigh. If your partner's lower leg is fleshy enough, continue across the outside of the knee and onto the calf. This stroke blends easily with the percussion movements you used on the back. Add them here for variety if your partner is a percussion fan.

♦ Spend extra time on the final two front-of-the-legs strokes: ten repetitions instead of the usual three. If you decide to extend clapping to the ankle, consider adding a small pillow just under the knee to elevate the side of the joint and make it easier to massage. Clapping and full-body stroking conclude both the fluid release effect on the legs as well as the entire massage of the lower half of your partner's body.

End massage of your first leg with clapping, then grasp your partner's opposite calf with one hand and start on the other leg. Cross over to the opposite side of her body while maintaining a light, even contact on the calf. Take your time when changing sides. Be careful not to lean forward onto your partner's leg while you move. After clapping on the second leg, do the full-body stroke that follows.

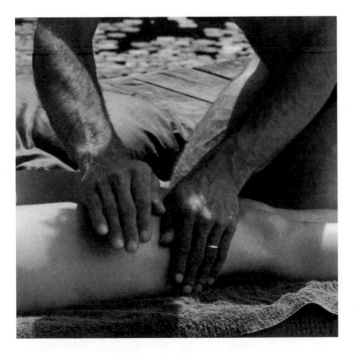

Full-Body Circulation

The lymph system removes acidic irritants and toxins from the body's tissues. But since it has no heart of its own, the system depends on local muscle contraction to move fluids from the extremities to collect in central nodes. Unfortunately, the chemicals that cause stress — lactic and carbonic acid, concentrations of nitrogen and salt — freeze the muscles, causing them to clamp down on the tiny lymph channels and eventually the vascular system itself. Witness the bloodless complexion of stressed individuals. Fluid release massage breaks this cycle of stress by pushing chemical irritants out of the muscles while oxygenating the whole body. This cleansing effect, more than anything else, produces the incomparable high that lingers for days after a full-body massage.

Complete your leg massage with a great tactile drum roll, a crescendo of sensation that sweeps from one end of the body to the other. With a single lavish two-hand sequence, your partner's entire body is enveloped in a wave of pure sensual pleasure. If you need one stroke to convert a hesitant individual to the joys of massage, choose this one.

During this stroke, your hands follow a mirror image of the full-body movement you used at the end of the back massage. Oil the front and sides of your partner's legs and chest (to the neck) before you begin. Start with your palms down, fingers wrapped around the front of your partner's ankles. As always, make contact from the tips of your fingers to the base of your palms. Your hands will move up and down the body together.

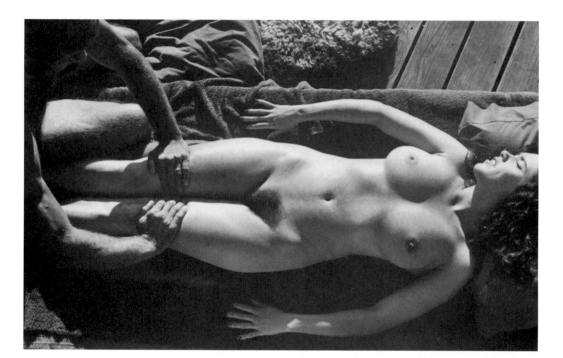

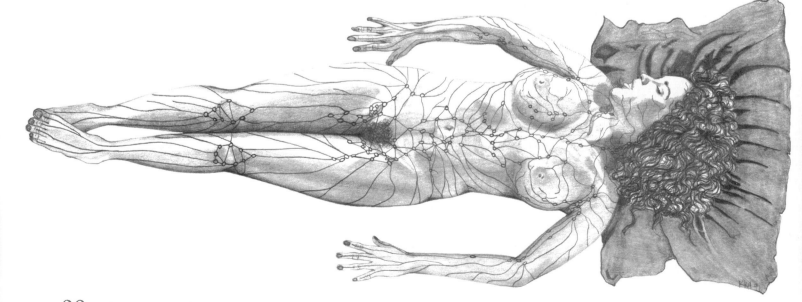

Press forward on both legs over the top of the knees and onto the hips. Move up the legs, repositioning yourself at the hips as you massage. Turn your hands so the fingertips nearly brush while continuing up across the chest. Turn them again at the top of the chest — stay off the throat — and move out over the shoulder tops. Rotate around the shoulder tops to the armpits. From that point on the top sides of the chest, pull straight down the side of the body all the way to the ankles. Keep your fingers together as you pull.

Reposition yourself, once again, as quietly as possible, when you cross the waist. Turn your hands a final time at the ankles and return to the starting position. Don't rush the final turn — your partner will notice. Repeat the whole sequence three times — ten times or more if you feel generous.

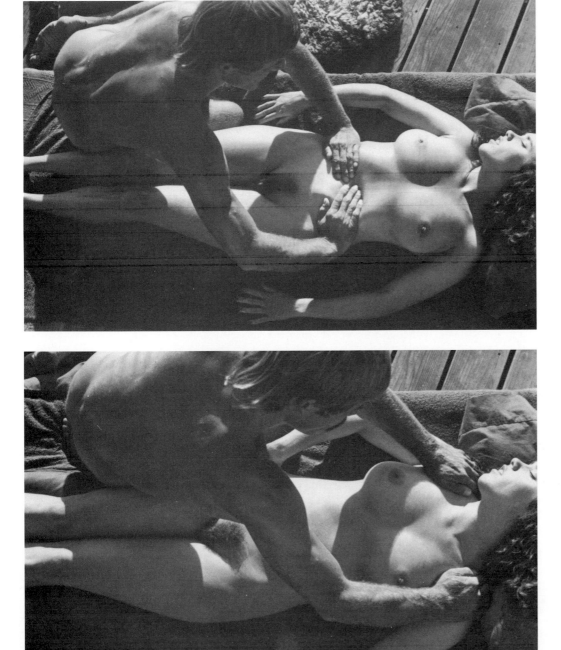

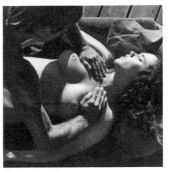

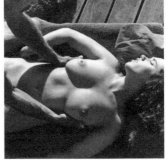

CHAPTER 8

The Chest

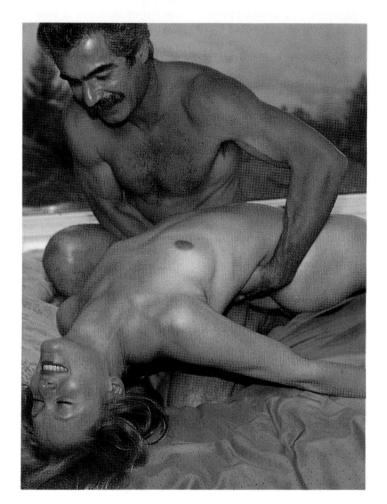

The legs gave you a chance to work the flesh with penetrating kneading and friction movements that nobody can resist. Can you continue with more of the same above the waist? If the arms look promising, the bony surface of the chest seems to offer little opportunity for any kind of deep massage. It's tempting to stroke the chest a few times and hurry on to the arms. Actually, the chest is much more than a convenient bridge between the fleshy legs and the arms; it signals the beginning of a gentler approach to your partner's body.

For the most part, after crossing the waist, you will abandon deep pressure strokes for the rest of the massage. From now on, go easy wherever you encounter soft fleshy areas, like below the rib cage or near the neck. Here, penetrating strokes like the ones you used on the heavily muscled portions of the legs and back will disturb internal structures.

assage derives its great power partly from its ability to liberate the body's largest organ, the skin. Like the back, the chest offers great expanses of skin that can be massaged in a single stroke. Forever wrapped in fabric and shielded from human contact, the chest has been starved for touch, perhaps since childhood. Massage lets the skin take its place at the center of the sensual world. The effects spread gradually, through tiny subcutaneous muscles, all over the chest. Glance at your partner's face during chest massage. You may notice the smile of deep relaxation and pleasure that only massage can bring.

The chest is also your window to the vital organs and the central nodes of the lymph system, the body's most important cleansing mechanism. With direct nerve paths that sweep straight around the body from the spine, the whole area from the waist to the shoulders is exquisitely sensitive. The strokes that follow leave your partner feeling as though a long-forgotten need has finally been fulfilled.

◆ Chest massage puts you face to face with your partner. Be silent. Let your hands say it.

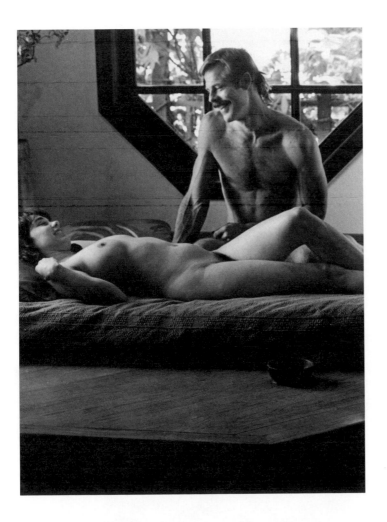

Full-Hand Stroking

Begin this luxurious full-hand stroke with your hands together, thumbs touching on the center of your partner's stomach (as shown). Using light to moderate pressure, press forward with one hand while you pull straight back with the other. Curve your fingers to fit against the sides of your partner's body. Push one hand forward while pulling the other back, until the fingertips of one hand and the heel of the other brush the massage surface on opposite sides of the body. Then reverse the movement, pulling your hands around to the far sides of the abdomen. Always let your fingers mold themselves to the changing shape of your partner's body. As you stroke back and forth, move up the abdomen and across the chest to the shoulder tops.

Stroke up and back to the shoulders three times. Use less pressure and extra oil over a woman's breasts but be sure to include them. Attempting to massage around the breasts will needlessly interrupt the stroke and cheat your partner. Full-hand stroking warms half of the body and leaves your partner feeling good from neck to hips.

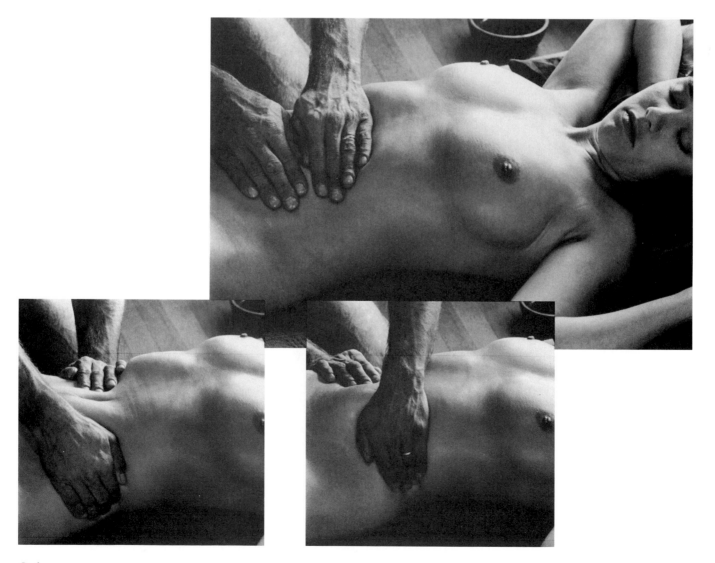

Pressing the Digestive Tract

To reduce tension on the muscles of the abdomen, elevate your partner's knees with a pillow during this stroke. Your fingertips will trace the semicircular course of the large digestive tract from its starting point just below the left side of the rib cage. Reach across from the right side of your partner's body; the stroke becomes awkward if you try it from the left side.

Starting from the top left side of the abdomen and ending on the top right, make a three-quarter circle with the fingertips of your right hand. You don't need much pressure; press down just hard enough to make a noticeable depression in the flesh. When you reach the end of the

U-shaped pattern, begin the same stroke with your left hand. As your left hand completes the stroke, start again with your right hand. Moving at the same moderately slow speed, the hands follow close behind each other. Complete the whole two-hand cycle ten times, pressing down with your fingertips (as shown).

Pressing enhances the digestive process and soothes the involuntary muscles of the abdomen. Just beneath your hands, bits of undigested food and debris shake loose from the walls of the digestive tract. Blood circulation in tiny capillaries is stimulated. These subtle internal changes may go unnoticed during the massage but the effects stay with your partner long afterward.

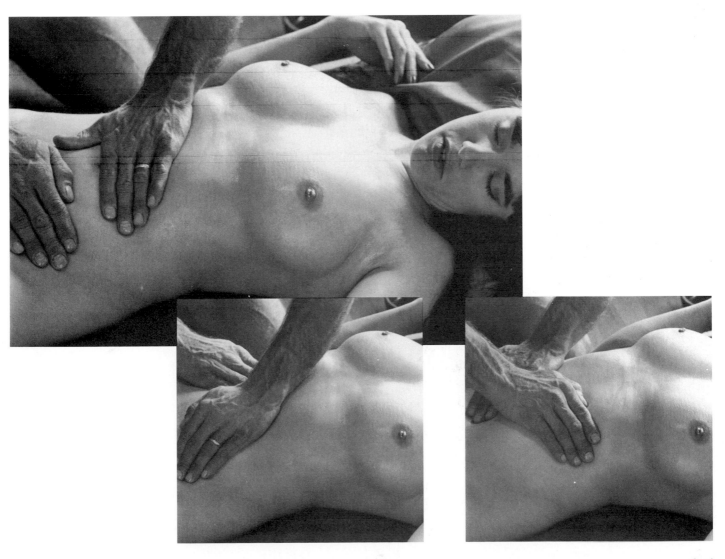

The Waist Lift

One of the most beautiful strokes in massage, more like dance than passive exercise, the waist lift makes both of you feel good. While flexing the lower back, it trains your partner's body to lean back and simply surrender to relaxation. Do the lift while facing either your partner's head or her feet — both variations are shown here. Facing the head, you will get a better grip on the lower back; turned to face the feet, you can grasp the lower part of the rib cage.

Reach through the hollow of your partner's back and lace your fingers together over the spine. Lift with the full surface of your hands, spreading the pres-

sure as evenly as possible across the lower back. If necessary, to gain more leverage while lifting, you may want to kneel on one knee (that is, kneel on one knee with your opposite foot flat on the floor to brace yourself) before you start. Pull straight up, lifting her lower back off the massage surface until you feel resistance — usually between six to twelve inches high. Hold the lift at the top position for a few moments, then let the back down slowly — a sudden drop will shock your partner. After returning her back to the full flat position, lift again. Repeat the stroke three times, moving at the same deliberate speed throughout the lifting and lowering.

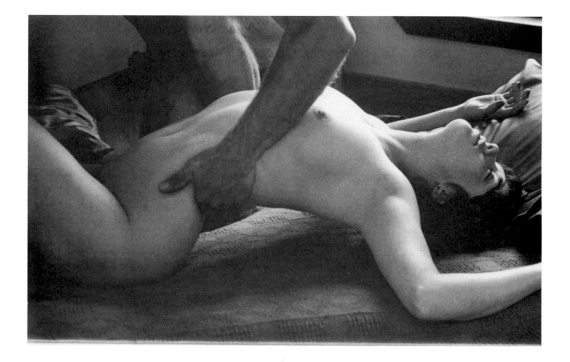

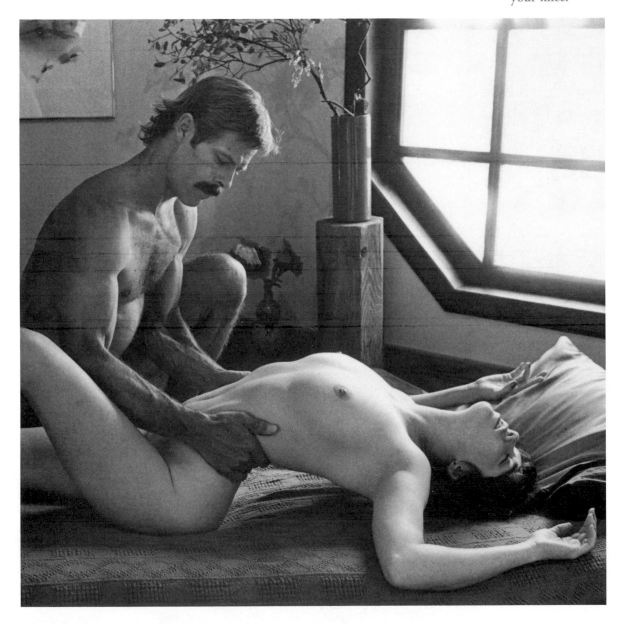

Kneading the Side of the Body

Knead your partner's side from the hips to the armpits, back and forth, at least three times. Use the full surface of your hands from one end of the body to the other. Near the hips, use your thumbs to pick up a fold of skin with each kneading stroke (as shown), but don't force the flesh up if you feel resistance. Over the ribs this stroke becomes a flat-fingered kind of kneading during which the hands move in the usual full circles without actually picking up any flesh. Either way, the stroke relaxes and tones muscles up and down the side of the body.

Knead slowly; let your partner feel the surface of your hands rotating in rhythmic circles up and down her side.

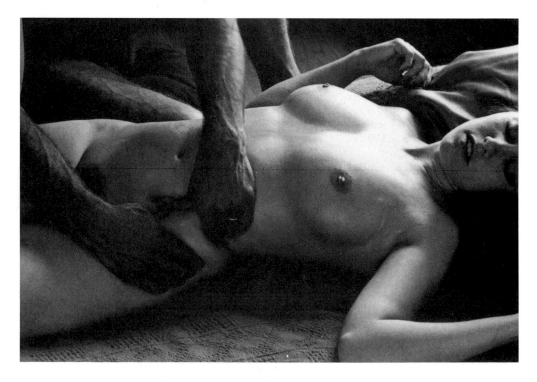

Full-Hand Friction

The external obliques, the wrap-around muscles of the back and abdomen, also respond well to a few minutes of restrained full-hand friction — too much pressure will disturb the kidneys. Combined with full-hand kneading, this stroke thoroughly relaxes the whole side of the body. Use friction over knotted muscles, then knead generously until you feel the last traces of tension melt.

Reach across from the opposite side of your partner's body, open your thumb wide on the anchor hand, and press into the gap with four fingers of the other hand (as shown). Circle with the full surface of your hand while pressing in with your fingertips. Move up the side of the chest, but go easy on the ribs.

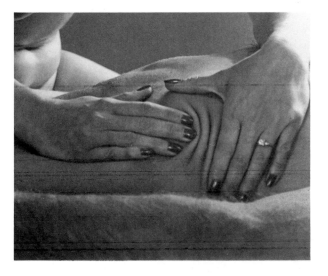

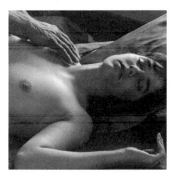

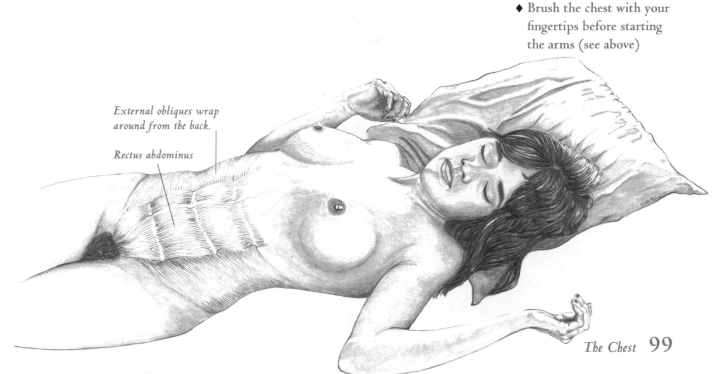

External obliques wrap around from the back.

Rectus abdominus

Chest and Shoulder Friction

Chest friction works on two levels: a fingertip version reaches deep within the muscular shoulder joint, while a lighter full-hand variation stimulates lymph flow in the cluster of nodes just below the shoulder.

On the shoulder: During friction strokes, the shoulder will move away from your hand unless the joint is well supported. Anchor the stroke by sliding one hand beneath your partner's back (as shown) and grasping the shoulder from below. Like so many purely mechanical aids to massage, the extra support feels surprisingly good. Who knows when your partner's shoulder was last properly caressed? Raise her shoulder slightly to meet your friction hand. Press down into the joint with your fingertips as you move around the muscular shoulder in small, even circles.

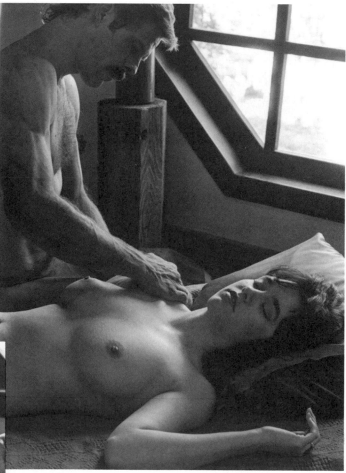

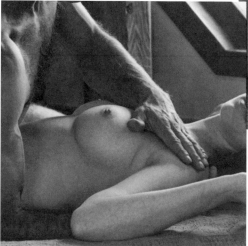

On the chest: Mold your hands to the changing shape of your partner's chest. Press down with the whole surface of your hand and rotate slowly, putting a bit of extra pressure on your fingertips. Spend extra time on the area just above the armpit where the lymph nodes that drain the breast are concentrated (as shown).

Chest friction travels easily. Reach up over the top of the shoulder to circle against the thick muscles on the back of the neck, but stay off the front and side of the neck.

Pause for a moment before massaging the irregular combination of muscle and bone at the shoulder. Circle lightly over the joint with your fingertips, noting the location of major bones. During shoulder friction you must pass over bony areas, but reserve the pressure part of each stroke for obviously muscular tissue. Circle right up to the point where muscle and bone join without actually pressing on the bone itself. If your partner has muscular upper arms, press down hard just below the shoulder joint.

The intricate lymph network of the female breast, one of the most complex anywhere on the body, is drained by a concentration of nodes around the armpit. Extra fingertip friction here helps clear the system. You don't have to press hard or dig in — the nodes are just beneath the surface. Using light pressure, circle with the flat surface of your fingertips.

During this stroke, you may want to move your partner's arm until her hand is over the top of her head. Never pull the arm from the wrist, a breach of massage etiquette. Use both hands to provide support above and below the elbow, whenever you move an arm.

Lift and carry her body. Hold it. Each little tactile courtesy will please your partner.

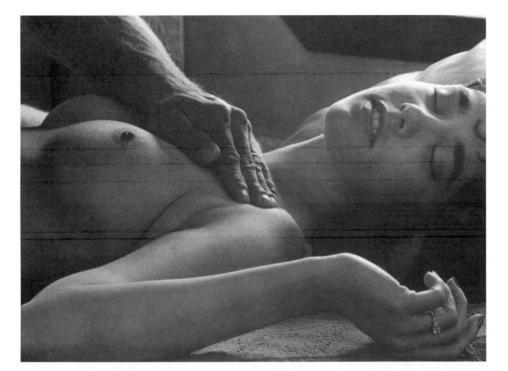

Lymph system and nodes

Vibrating the Chest

One of the most satisfying chest movements works from the opposite side of the body. While sitting above your partner's shoulder tops, slide your hands straight down beneath the upper back. Lift straight up against the back of the rib cage with both hands and move your fingers up and down for half a minute. Her chest will vibrate above your hands. Use this movement as a prelude to direct percussion strokes over the lungs.

Chest Thumping

Few strokes in massage have a more immediate effect inside the body than chest thumping. This is a crucial stress-control stroke simply because it reaches right through to the body's vital organs. Thumping gets your partner thinking about massage and pleasure instead of dwelling on his problems. But the stroke also has a way of bringing massage to parts of the body most other movements cannot reach. Use it here to oxygenate the heart and lungs.

The stroke works the same way here that it did on the back (see page 47). Strike the back of one hand with your closed fist. Be sure to break each downward motion at the wrist. A light tapping travels back and forth across the rib cage, loosening debris in the lungs and increasing oxygen levels in the blood. Your partner will feel this stroke right through the thickest part of his body. A palpable feeling of lightness and energy floods the body after just a few minutes of chest thumping.

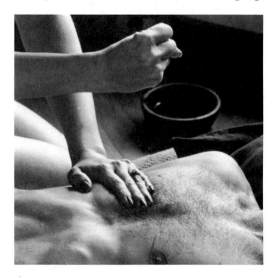

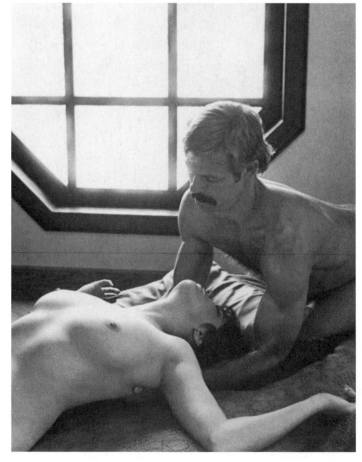

Half-Body Stroking

A great favorite with women, half-body stroking covers more skin surface than any other chest stroke — from the shoulders to the waist (or as far down as you can reach comfortably on the torso), as well as both sides of the body and parts of the back. Use it to warm the entire trunk of the body one final time before you move off the chest onto the arms.

Kneel or sit above your partner's head. Oil the chest, sides and upper back before you begin. Lift each one of your partner's shoulders with one hand and spread oil under it with the other. Press the heels of your hands against your partner's shoulders, your fingers pointed toward the waist (as shown). Keeping your fingers together, stroke straight ahead to the waist. Use light pressure over the breasts. When you reach the waist, move your hands apart until you are grasping the sides of the body (as shown). Pull straight up the sides, bending your hands in under your partner's shoulder blades. When

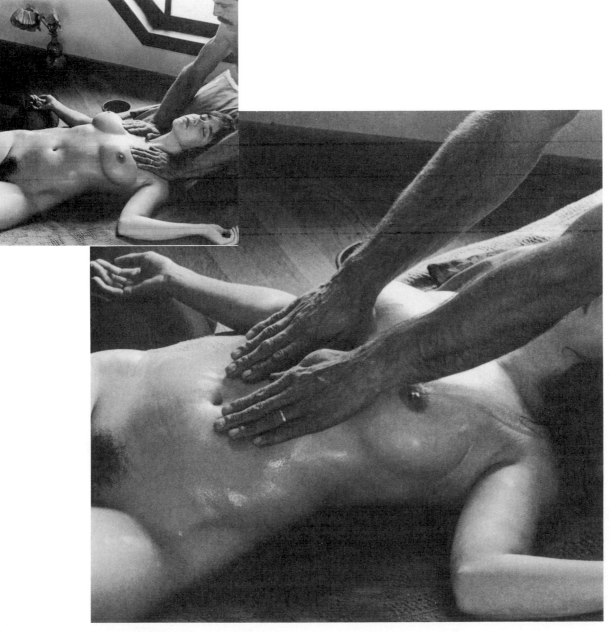

WRAP-AROUND SENSATION ZONES

This half-body movement, one of the sleeper strokes in massage, provides tactile delights far beyond the obvious. It feels so good because you're stroking across more than a dozen sensation zones that are connected directly to the spine. You can be certain your partner will experience deep pleasure every inch of the way. Glance at her face while you pull up the back. She's tracking your hands.

you feel the rib cage above your hands, press up with your fingers. Lift the chest as you pull up toward the shoulders. Turn your hands again at the shoulders and return to the starting position.

Throughout the first few sequences pay extra attention to oiling, especially during the lifting portion of the stroke. Be prepared to add more oil if you feel your hands pulling against your partner's

skin. Try the whole movement a few times slowly until the stroking, pulling, and lifting motions flow together. Then move a bit faster, using the same moderate speed on both sides of the body. Get it right and your partner will experience a wave of delicious sensation that flows down the chest, up the sides, and finally lifts half the body before returning to the shoulder tops.

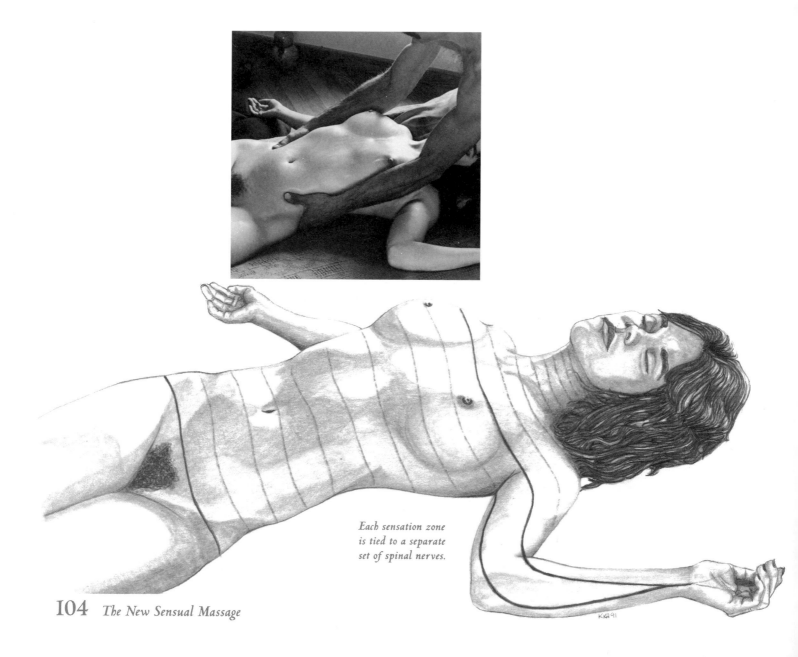

Each sensation zone is tied to a separate set of spinal nerves.

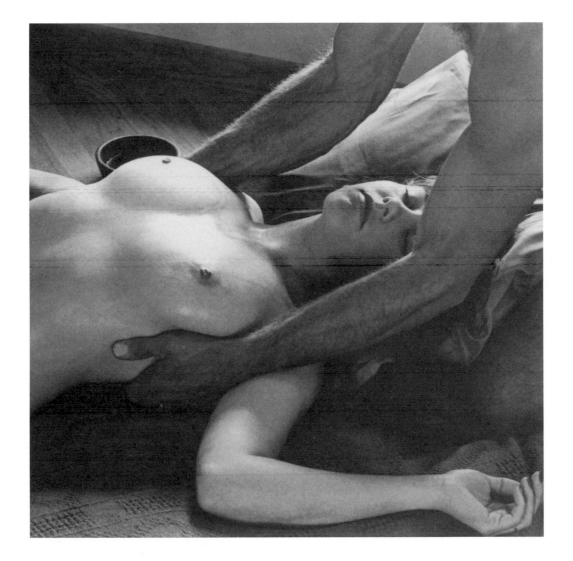

CHAPTER 9

The Arms

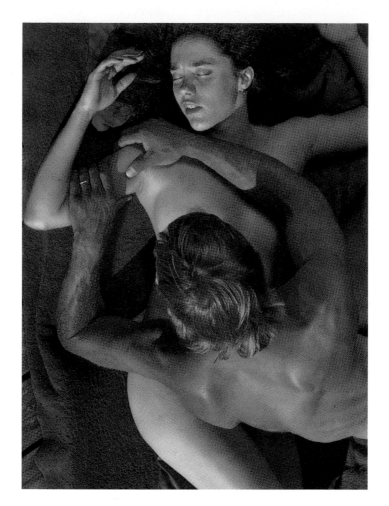

Just when computers were beginning to make life easier it turned out that the added efficiency had a hidden price tag: carpal tunnel syndrome (see page 123). This repetitive strain injury, the bane of the computer revolution, can leave your partner unable to use his hands without experiencing great pain. But this is not a uniquely modern problem: A hundred years ago masseurs went to great lengths to develop a treatment for a condition then known as "writer's cramp," which produced paralyzing pain in the hands and arms of clerical workers. Actually, it makes little difference whether you use a quill pen or computer: The pain is caused by hour after hour of close repetitive work with the fingers in an unfriendly environment — like relentless telephone dialing or data processing while sitting in a confined, inflexible workstation.

Think of the nerves of the arms as wires from the body to the hands. Put too much pressure on the wires and the hands stop working properly. The three main nerves of the arm — ulnar, radial, and median — which originate in the neck, are vulnerable to pressure in two spots: the infamous carpal ligament of the wrist (more on that in the next chapter) and the top joint of the arm where all three nerves bend sharply under the pectoralis minor, an interior chest muscle. It's best to relax the muscles of the arm first, before hand massage, to take pressure off the whole length of these nerves. Arm strokes also relax the tendons of the forearm that operate the hand.

The arms are massaged from the bottom — here, the wrist — up, somewhat like the legs. But since the arms are thinner, it doesn't take much massage to temporarily dilate the capillaries and produce a tangible feeling of warmth. After a few dozen circulation and kneading movements, you begin to see a change in the skin. The reddish blush will fade but the skin comes away from arm massage softer and more supple, with a healthy glow.

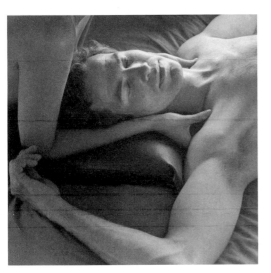

Many headaches originate in pinched nerves around the shoulder area.

When the pectoralis minor, an interior muscle near the shoulder (shown below), is stressed, it tugs directly on the nerve bundle that supplies the arm and hand. But tightness here also puts pressure on the nerves that supply the head, which originate under the shoulder blade. Because it's not visible on the surface of the body, it's tempting to skip over this extremely sensitive spot; many masseurs do.

You have massaged the shoulders as part of the back massage, and you'll do it again as part of relaxing the head and working on the arms.

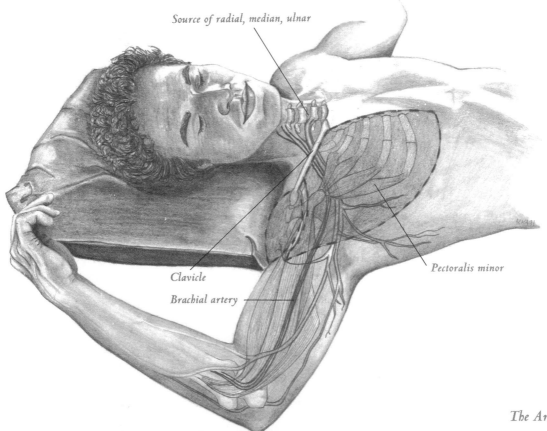

Source of radial, median, ulnar

Clavicle

Brachial artery

Pectoralis minor

♦ If your partner has long hair, gently use one hand to move it off her shoulders; remember to move the hair with as much care as you would use on a limb. Then, oil the arm you're about to massage from the wrist to the shoulder. Press the oil forward with long, flat-hand motions that will complement the stroke itself.

Circulation

Pressing the blood toward the heart through the large surface veins of the arms warms the chest and invigorates the arms. Do this stroke twice during arm massage: once at the outset and again, to enhance the fluid release effect, just before you move off the arms and onto the hands.

Circulation works the same way on the arms as on the legs. With your fingers pressed together, cup your hands around your partner's wrist. As you move forward, both your fingertips and the heel of your hands should touch the massage surface.

Press up toward the shoulder, keeping your fingers wrapped around the sides of the arm. You will feel a roll of flesh just ahead of your little finger. Turn at the shoulder just as you did at the hip, allowing one hand to sweep up over the top of the joint, in this case the shoulder, while the other turns sharply into the armpit. The two hands descend along the sides of the arm opposite each other, making light contact. Without breaking contact, turn your hands again at the wrist and return to the starting position. Ten times up and down the arm with this stroke leaves your partner feeling warm and relaxed.

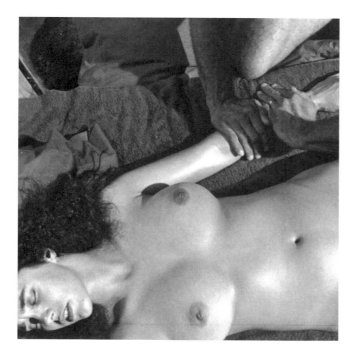
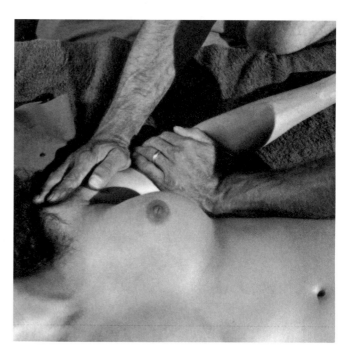

Hand-Over-Hand Pulling

Since the arms are shorter than the legs, it's always tempting to extend the longer strokes by reversing them at the shoulder. Go ahead; your partner will thank you. This combination provides a kind of high-intensity massage with waves of pleasing sensation flowing in both directions up and down the whole length of the arm.

Use both hands to lift your partner's arm, supporting it above and below the elbow. Grasp the arm close to the armpit with one hand and place the other hand just below it. Pull straight down, first with one hand, then the other. This is a fast, hand-over-hand stroke that begins by concentrating on a few inches of the arm, then expands. Move past the elbow one hand at a time so the arm doesn't drop suddenly. After a few repetitions, change to a long, pulling variation that covers the whole arm. When you reach the wrist area, begin longer full-arm strokes that extend from the armpit to the wrist — use the greatest distance that's comfortable for you. It's fun to move back and forth between the long and short variations of arm pulling.

EXTRA OIL

◆ Expect plenty of contact during hand-over-hand pulling on the arms. During this stroke, your fingers wrap around to the elbow side, while your thumbs ride on the muscular top. The down stroking motion is vigorous and repetitive — you may need extra oil.

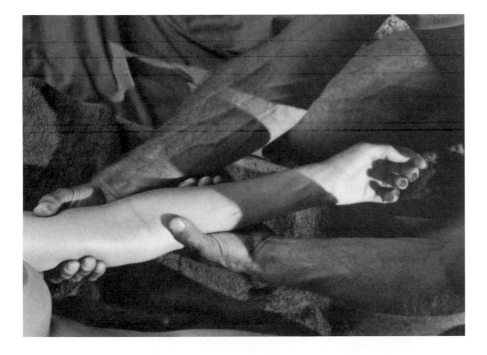

Knuckle Compression

The thick muscles of the upper arm follow an irregular path from the shoulder to the elbow. Most strokes that massage them are broken into two sections: one for the shoulder, another for the upper arm. The trick here, during knuckle compression, is to follow the whole course of the muscles while pressing down moderately hard — without contacting the bone.

First, to establish the path of the stroke, trace the muscles with your fingertips starting on the fleshy part of the shoulder and curving around to the top of the arm. Knuckle pressing starts on the shoulder and moves down close to the elbow. At the start, anchor the movement on the middle of the arm.

Press the flat part of your knuckle against the fleshy fold of muscle on the top of your partner's shoulder and circle slowly. Move around to the side of the shoulder, then down onto the top central muscles of the upper arm, the biceps. As you move toward the elbow, reposition your anchor hand over the wrist. This keeps the forearm in place while you apply compression to the muscles near the elbow. Circling with your fingertips, move up and down the arm. Reposition your anchor hand to keep your partner's arm still, whenever necessary.

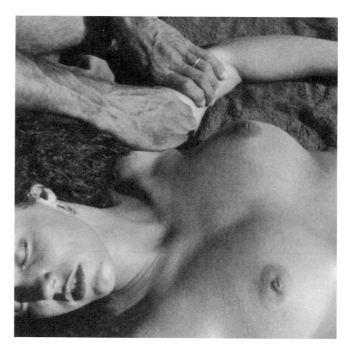

Shoulder Kneading

Knead the shoulder's small but muscular top with your fingertips — use your full hand on large, muscular shoulders. Reach in and feel for the muscles. Unless your partner is exceedingly thin, you will be able to pick up a generous fold of tissue with each kneading stroke. However, if the muscles are tight, don't force them up lest you pinch the shoulder. Press down into the tightness with your fingertips.

Like fingertip kneading strokes elsewhere on the body, this movement travels well to adjoining structures, in this case, the whole top of the arm. Stay on the same muscles you massaged with compression. Pick up a fold of flesh with the fingers of one hand while the other hand opens wide. Circle as you knead.

Combine extra hand-over-hand pulling strokes with knuckle compression and shoulder kneading and, after awhile, the arms begin to radiate a healthy glow.

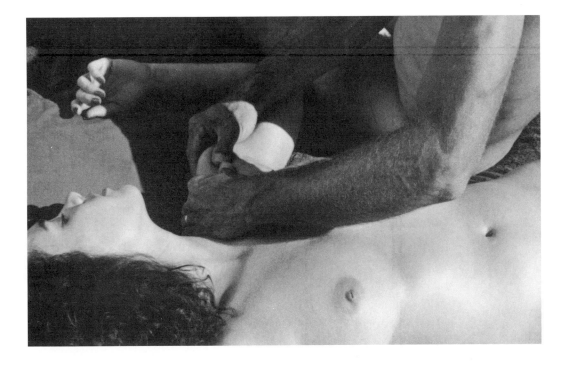

♦ Your partner's hand fits perfectly under your armpit. Make use of connections like that whenever you can. Massage is contact; everyone welcomes the feeling of being held.

Thumb Kneading the Arm

Knead the arm either on the massage surface or against your body. Elevating the arm to knead it brings you closer to your partner, establishing a body-to-body connection that is rare outside of massage. Gently clamp your partner's fingers under your armpit but allow the thumb to point up on the outside (as shown). Lifting the arm straight up, rest your partner's elbow on your knee. Now you have three body-to-body contact points: the armpit, the knee, and your hands.

Start by grasping the arm near the armpit and wrapping your fingers around the biceps. Press your thumbs down into those muscles and begin the thumb kneading stroke you used on the legs: the thumbs make small circles, rotating in opposition to each other. Descending slowly, massage the arm from the shoulder to the wrist, taking care not to press on the area above the elbow joint where large blood vessels are near the surface. Broaden your kneading on the forearm to include the whole surface of your thumbs from ball to tip.

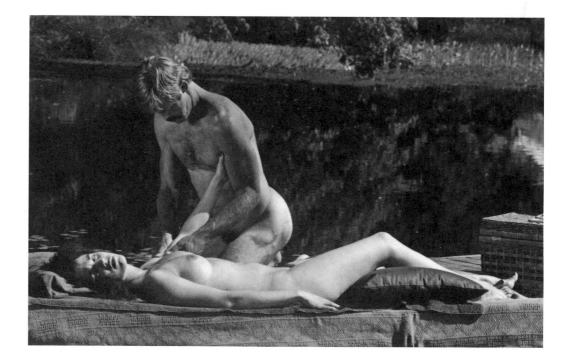

Kneading on the massage surface is just as effective, if a bit less personal. The stroke works the same way — simply grasp your partner's arm around the biceps and knead down the arm. Lift the arm a bit to slide your fingers down.

To prepare for hand massage, few strokes are more effective than kneading the forearm. Since the nerves and blood vessels of the arm supply the hand, kneading spreads benefits far beyond the immediate area. However, once you pass below the elbow, where the tendons that operate the hands originate, nearly everything you do directly enhances massage of the hands. Extra time spent kneading the forearm — for instance, ten repetitions, instead of the usual three — pays off on the hands.

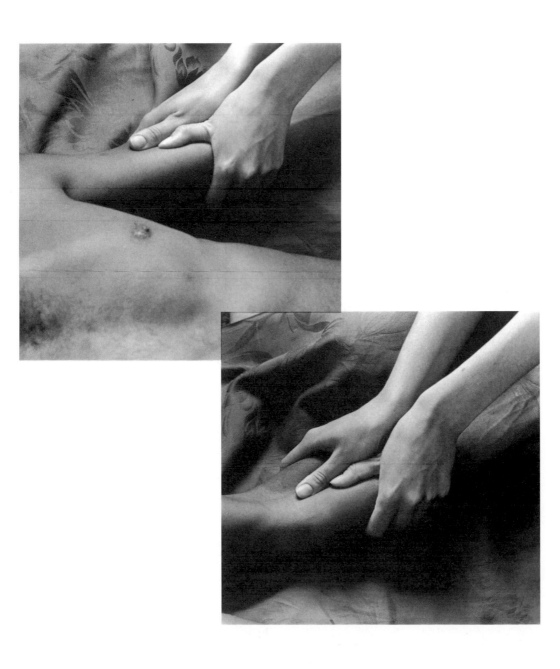

Elbow Friction

Consider elbow friction an optional but important stroke. The complex joint at the elbow, perhaps the most unusual anywhere in the body, is best massaged from your partner's opposite side. Instead of awkwardly moving across your partner's body just to do one stroke, reach over the chest and do elbow friction on the opposite arm (as shown).

Anchor the stroke by grasping your partner's arm just below the elbow. Start fingertip friction with the other hand just above the elbow and move down across the joint itself. Don't press in with your fingertips — major blood vessels lie just beneath the surface — rather, apply friction with the flat surface of your fingers. You'll feel the irregular elbow joint and the ends of the radius and ulna, the long bones of the forearm that cross over each other when the hand turns sharply.

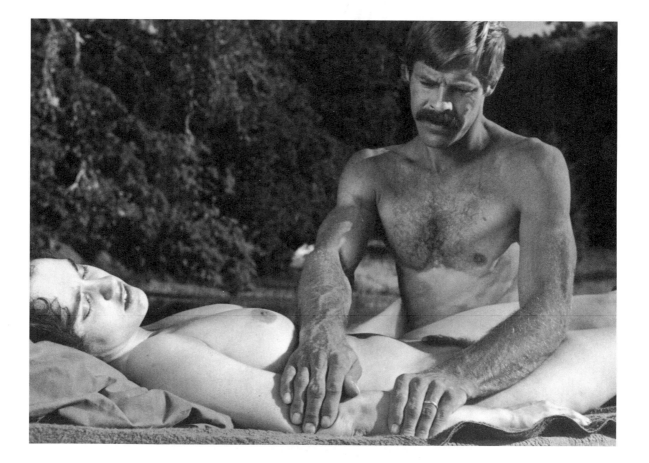

Passive Exercise Sequences

Think of the arms as your last, best chance to have fun with passive exercise, and use these strokes to make the most of it. Head massage, which comes next, is by comparison a sedate affair because the head likes it that way — the neck and jaws have a limited range of movement. The arms, however, can move in huge arcs at two different joints. These movements send your partner's arms flying through the air, an exuberant climax to your passive exercise routines elsewhere on the body.

Your partner will delight in the anti-gravity effects and the feeling of controlled abandon — but it's up to you to maintain control. Get sloppy and your partner's arm will crash-land against your chest or, worse, onto the massage surface. That will bring the massage to a sudden halt and your partner bolt upright.

Now you're ready to move the arm in some truly interesting ways, as you'll see in the six passive exercise sequences that follow.

Carpal ligament

Radius ulna crossing

Humerus

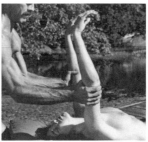

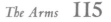

◆ Before you start, you might want to remind your partner not to help you lift the arms. You do all the work in a passive exercise sequence; she does nothing at all.

Rotating the Forearm

Start your passive exercise routine by rotating just half the arm from the elbow. You've got to take off before you can fly.

To limit the effects to the forearm, anchor the stroke above the elbow; wrap your fingers around your partner's arm while pressing down gently (as shown). Then, grasp your partner's arm at the wrist, lift straight up and rotate it in wide circles outward from the waist. The inside of the circle will pass over your partner's abdomen. Actually, the precise shape of the "circle," determined by the irregular joint at the elbow, may be almost ellipti-

cal. As in all passive exercise movements, feel for the point of tension and rotate just inside.

Do three conservative rotations, while keeping the hand bent forward. Follow with three more, widening the circle just enough to let your partner's hand bend back at the wrist by itself while turning. This accommodation allows you to take full advantage of the strange and wonderful architecture of the lower arm. As the hand turns, the bones in the forearm will cross, making for smoother and wider circles.

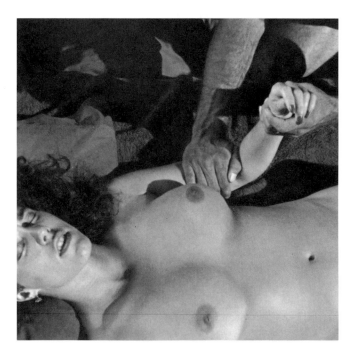

Rotating the Shoulder

By gripping the shoulder firmly from above and below, you can rotate the whole joint in tiny circles. Slide one hand under the shoulder and cup the top of the joint with your other hand (as shown). Before turning your hands, lift the shoulder straight up and move it back and forth to feel the various points of tension. Lift from below as you press down from above. Rotate your partner's shoulder in small circles just inside the points of tension. Turn three times in each direction, then gently lower the shoulder to the massage surface.

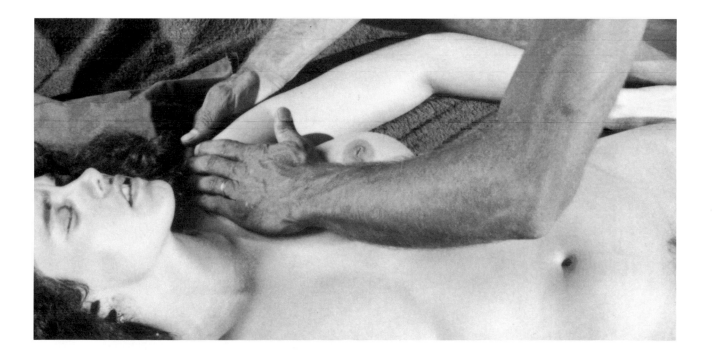

Squeezing the Arm

With this stroke, the whole arm rises straight up into the air, where it will stay for the next few minutes. Arm squeezing allows your partner to become comfortable with one of the most unusual situations in massage: You manipulate the whole arm while it remains perfectly relaxed in a vertical position.

Grasp your partner's arm at the wrist and lift it straight up. Squeeze the top and bottom of the arm (not the sides). Feel the biceps with your top fingers. Move up the arm, squeezing gently every few inches, until you touch your support hand at the wrist. Reverse the stroke there and return to the starting point. Three complete cycles and your partner will realize that we all need to have our arms squeezed from time to time.

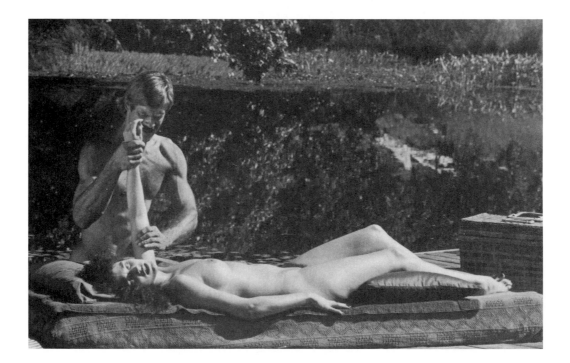

Rubbing the Arm

By now your partner is used to having you pick up and move her arm. Everything you've done so far has been pleasing and she's waiting to see what new adventures you have in store for her arm. This stroke won't disappoint her.

Lift the arm again, carefully, and fold her hand straight across the chest (as shown). Holding the arm in the folded position, press the flat part of both your hands against the sides of her upper arm. While continuing to press inward, rub the hands back and forth in a horizontal piston motion. As you rub, press up the arm.

Don't stop when you reach the elbow joint, simply continue your upward rubbing and the forearm will rise to meet your hands. Go up as far as the wrist and stop when her arm is fully extended. Reversing the movement can become awkward — better to start again from the top of the arm. Carefully fold your partner's arm and return to the starting point on the upper arm. Lower the arm into the same folded position you used at the outset. Don't rush arm rubbing — your hands should move back and forth about twice every second. Give your partner plenty of time to relish the new sensation.

Rubbing warms the whole arm and leaves your partner basking in a tangible physical glow.

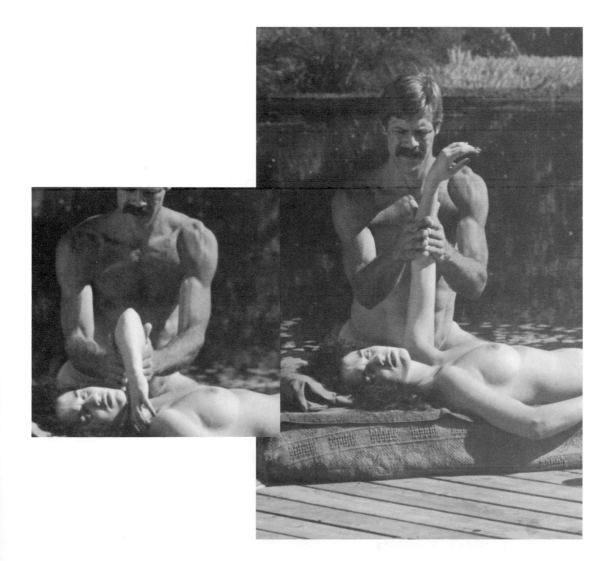

Flexing the Shoulders

Pulling on a limb exerts pressure on the joint directly above your hands. Use the arms as levers to pull and turn both massive shoulder joints while stretching out internal ligaments.

Kneel above your partner's head and grasp both arms just below the elbows. Lift straight up until the hands are vertical (as shown). Pull up and rotate the arms slowly. As the joint turns, you will feel a slight resistance; don't press beyond that point. Each time you stretch the internal ligaments and tendons of the shoulders, they become more supple. The next time you do this stroke, you will notice the difference — and so will your partner.

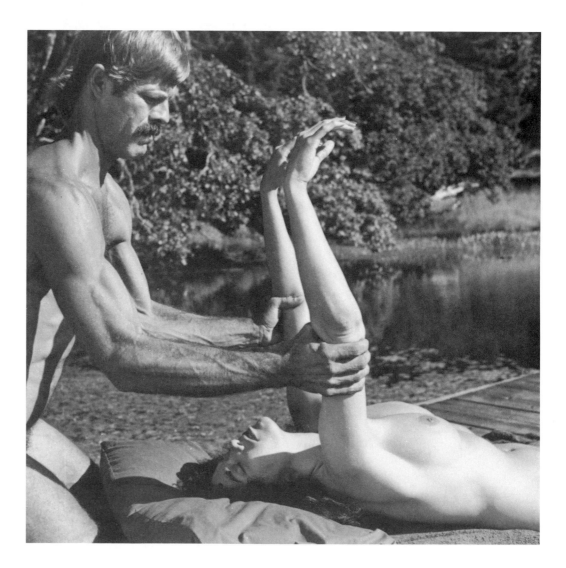

Tossing the Arms

During arm tossing, everyone's favorite passive exercise movement, the arms acquire a life of their own, happily sailing through the air with no help from your partner. Your arms have always wanted to do this.

Arm tossing shouldn't come as a surprise, lest it go out of control. Test the limits of the stroke first and show your partner what to expect. Pick up her arm, holding it loosely at the wrist, then toss it from one hand to another in a gentle arc no more than one foot long. At this point you're simply training her body to accept the tossing motion. As you catch the arm,

move your hand back to soften the impact. After a half dozen short practice tosses, you're ready to get serious.

Gradually widen the arc until you are catching your partner's hand well above the shoulder at one end and parallel to her leg at the other. As always, feel for the point of tension as the arm moves back and forth and massage just inside of it. Remember to move your hand with the arm each time you catch it. Start with a relaxed frequency — a throw every two seconds — and build up to two or three times a second. Arm tossing will leave your partner smiling. A thriller.

BRUSHING THE ARMS

◆ Abruptly ending arm massage after tossing can be unsettling. Add a gentle transition stroke to help your partner move from strong feelings up and down the arms to delicate ones on the hands.

Finish the arms with a hand-over-hand brushing stroke that begins on the shoulders, continues across the forearm, and ends on the back of the hand. Light contact with your fingertips will reach the interior nerves. Repeat three or four times.

End with long, unbroken movements from the shoulder to the wrist. Brushing makes an important tactile point: The sensation that has been focused on the arm now moves to the hand.

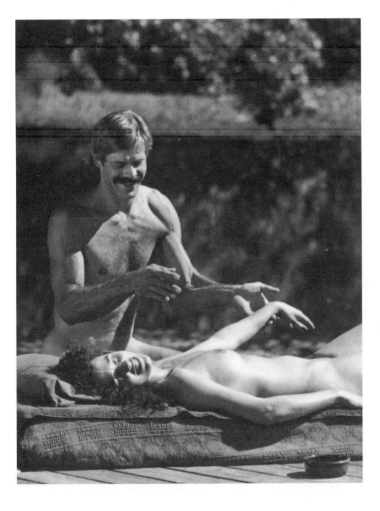

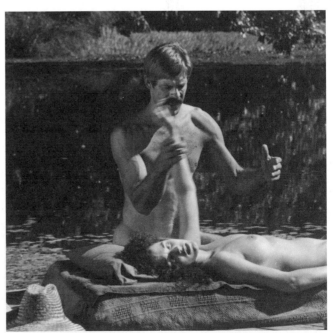

CHAPTER 10

The Hands

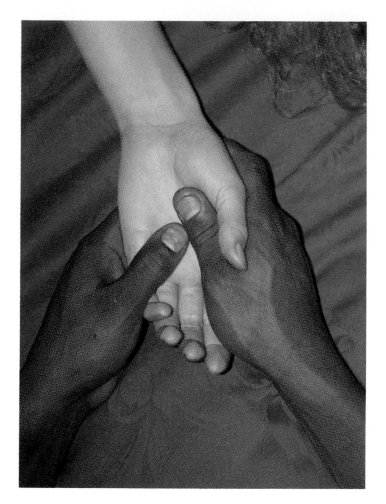

Thanks to the handshake, we're all accustomed to being touched on the hands. If your partner seems shy about being touched, stroke the hands before the next massage. This part of the full-body massage begins with a two-hand version of the familiar greeting, then moves on to explore some of the more interesting things hands can do for each other.

The hands are operated by remote control via long tendons and muscles that extend from the elbows. They merge, at the wrist, with a tight bundle of blood vessels and nerves and squeeze through a narrow joint capsule known as the carpal tunnel. The thick carpal ligament, which holds together the eight bones of the wrist, fits tightly around the whole bundle. If the hands are stressed, the tunnel contracts sharply, putting direct pressure on the same three major nerves of the arm that you first encountered at the shoulder: the ulnar, radial and, most vulnerable here, the median, which is pressed hard against the ligament itself.

Ligaments are tough ropelike fibers that connect one bone to another to form a joint. When a joint is twisted beyond its normal range, a few fibers of a supporting ligament may be torn or even ripped loose from the bone. Left to its own devices, the resulting injury, a sprain, heals slowly, because ligaments have notoriously poor blood supplies. As long ago as the American Civil War, however, medical professionals realized that the recovery time after a sprain could be reduced by half or more with regular massage of the affected area. Today we often use direct ligament massage to treat injuries like sprains.

The automated modern office hasn't been kind to the wrist joint. Scores of office workers are suffering from untreated carpal tunnel syndrome (CTS), a cumulative trauma disorder caused by repeated stressful movements of the hand and wrist. They experience a tingling and numbness that give way to pain so intense that ordinary tasks like writing or using kitchen utensils become difficult. We now know that ligament fibers at the wrist can be torn slowly through unaccustomed repetitive tasks, like typing on an awkward computer keyboard. Furthermore, with overuse, the synovial fluid that lubricates the tendon sheaths of the wrist and hand begins to diminish, causing friction, inflammation and more pain. If nothing is done to correct the problem, permanent joint pain and instability serve to remind the CTS victim how easily the human body can become the weak link in the chain of office automation.

Carpal ligament

Tendons of the hand

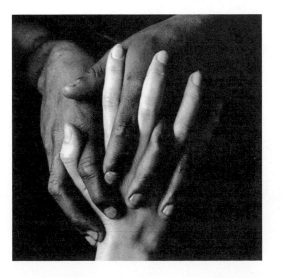

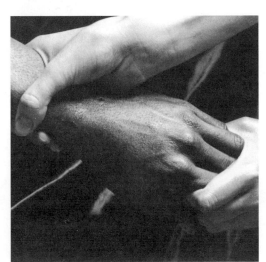

- Knead the extensor ten-
dons in the forearm first
- Support your partner's
arm at the elbow with a
pillow
- Don't press down on the
front of the wrist
- Massage the fingers on
both sides of the hand
- Pull up along the nerve-
rich sides of the fingers
- Massage the palm well
away from the legs
- Focus thumb kneading
on the base of the thumb
- Massage the back of the
hands next to the legs

Obviously, massage cannot repair a badly torn ligament, but by pumping oxygen-rich blood into the tissues, massage can speed the healing process. Better yet, a well-massaged hand and wrist will help to protect your partner from the ravages of CTS. Repeating a few simple movements in this chapter — thumb kneading the back and palm, knuckle pressing and rotating the hand — a dozen times or more will transform the oxygen-starved tissues of the wrist joint and leave your partner's hands feeling nearly weightless. Whether or not your partner is suffering from CTS, a thorough hand massage is a great pleasure. The hands deserve to feel good, so you can skip the therapeutic justification and just do it.

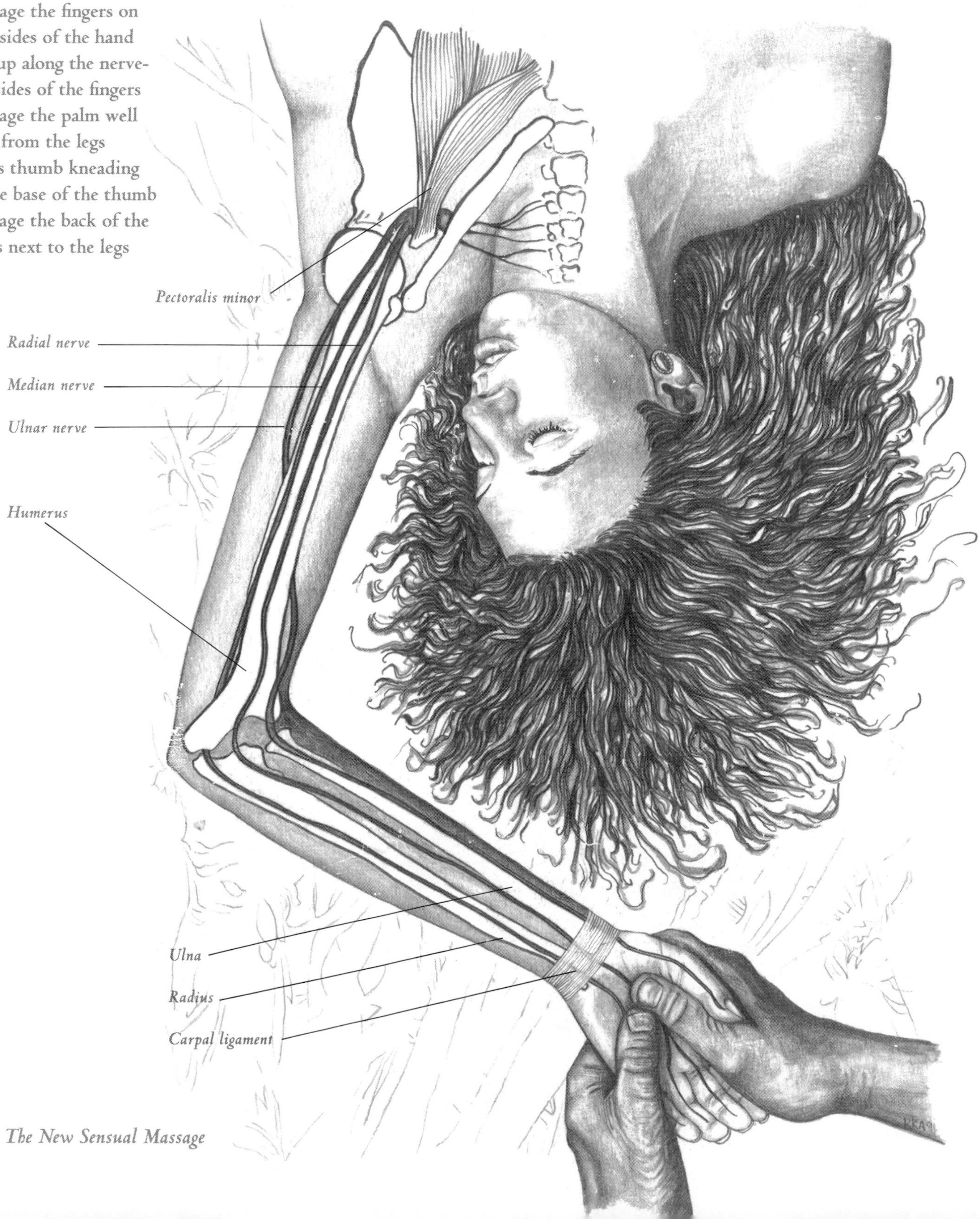

Pectoralis minor

Radial nerve

Median nerve

Ulnar nerve

Humerus

Ulna

Radius

Carpal ligament

Kneading the Palm

The three major nerves of the arm, the radial, ulnar, and median, emerge from the carpal tunnel and fan out across the palm. Palm kneading gives you an opportunity to massage them directly. Reach in with your thumbs to knead the irregular-shaped area from the base of the fingers to the wrist. Add a bit of extra oil to your partner's hand; you may want to support her arm at the elbow with a small pillow. Be generous with palm kneading, one of the most important strokes of the hand. Your thumbs fit conveniently into the depression of the palm, making this an easy movement to continue far beyond the usual three repetitions.

Using both of your hands, grasp the top of your partner's hand with your fingers while pressing inward against the palm with both thumbs. Rotate your thumbs — one up, while the other is down — making small circles against the soft inner tissues of the hand. The whole of the palm, especially around the base of the thumb, will accept more pressure than any other part of the hand. Press down until you begin to feel the bones beneath your thumbs. Pay special attention to the fleshy base of the thumb, but stay off the wrist itself, where large blood vessels are close to the surface.

Everyone relishes this stroke. A well-kneaded palm leaves the hand feeling strong and supple.

COMPUTER STRESS

◆ If your partner does close work with her fingers, like computer data entry, and has been experiencing discomfort around the hands and forearm, pay special attention to this stroke.

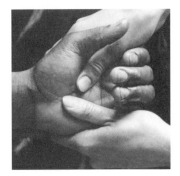

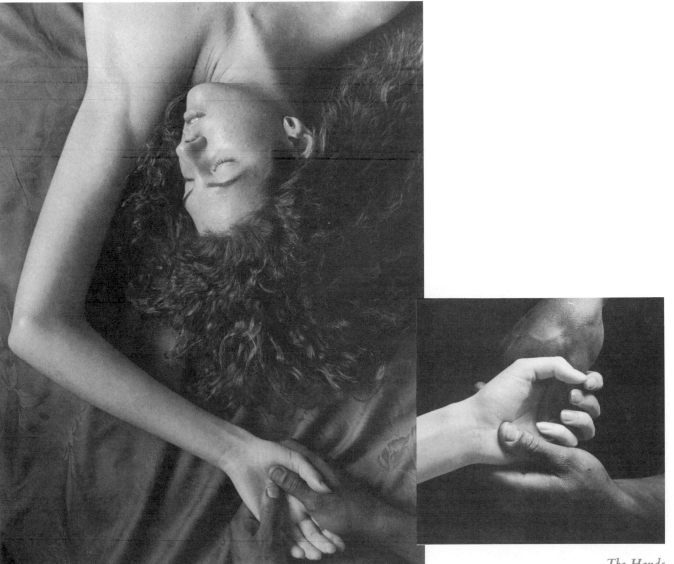

Knuckle Pressing the Palm

Knuckle pressing focuses deep pressure on your partner's open palm. To massage the center of the palm, hold her hand from below (as shown), make a fist and press straight down into the palm with the flat surface of your knuckles. First, rock your hand from side to side in the center of the palm, then rotate it in small circles as you press. Like palm kneading, this stroke travels slowly from the base of the palm to the bottom of the fingers.

To focus extra pressure on the fleshy heel of the hand, support your partner's hand below the wrist (as shown) before pressing down with your knuckles.

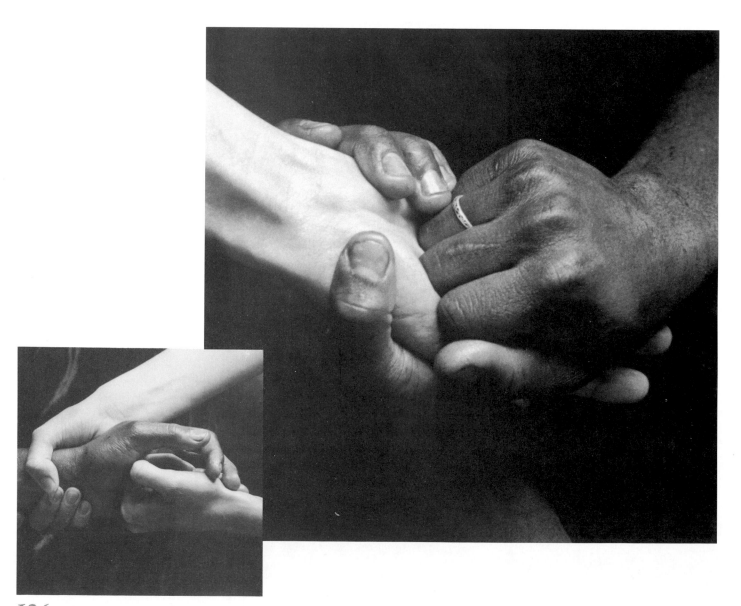

Turning Over the Hand

Due to the irregular joint at the elbow, when the palms are facing up, the hands will lie bent out as much as forty-five degrees from your partner's hip. The fingers point, quite naturally, away from the body while you massage the hand with the palms up. However, when you rotate the hand to massage the top side, the elbow joint straightens out, allowing your partner's hand to rest right next to her hip. Move closer to your partner's body for the next part of the hand massage.

Although the hand is the smallest body part you will massage, don't be tempted, during a rotation, to treat it with less consideration than a much larger limb. Support the hand across the wrist (as shown) then lift and rotate it slowly inward toward the body. Allow the elbow joint to adjust during this turn and the hand will fall comfortably where it wants to be, against the hip.

The back side of your partner's hand now faces straight up and awaits your massage.

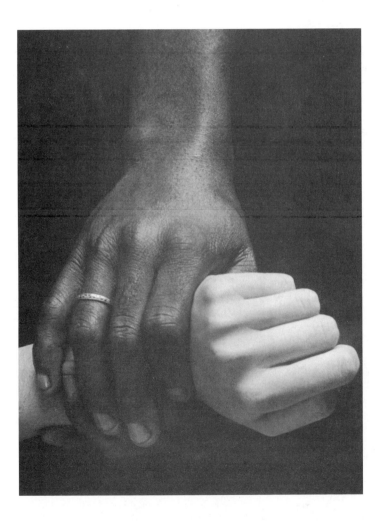

The Bone Roll

Using both of your hands, fold your fingers against your partner's palm and press your thumbs firmly against the top of the hand. Feel the tiny bones within. Time to move them.

Squeezing your fingertips against the base of your thumbs, gently rotate your hands forward, then back, in small circles. You will feel the bones begin to move with your hands.

Don't try to enlarge the circles. A little movement will give your partner yet another experience that cannot be had outside of massage: a soothing undulation through the whole hand; single-hand bone ripple — while the rest of the body relaxes.

Rotating the Hand

The hand turns in an irregular circle against the eight bones of the wrist joint. You'll feel the bones ripple quietly as you rotate the hand.

Grasp your partner's wrist with one hand and fold your other hand over the finger tops (as shown). While holding his wrist steady, use the fingers as a handle to rotate the hand. Go easy the first time around in order to feel the various points of resistance at the wrist. Turn the hand three times in each direction, working just inside the points of resistance.

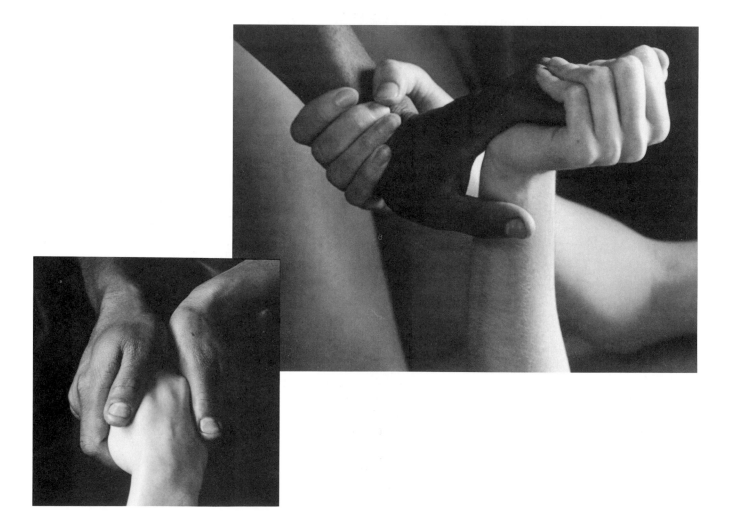

Flexing the Hand

Using both of your hands, grasp the top of your partner's hand with your fingers (as shown) and press up moderately hard against the palm with both thumbs. Pull outward across the top of the hand with your fingers while you continue to press up with your thumbs. You'll feel the bones again; this time you're simply flexing them outward. Three times feels good, six feels great.

Finger Flexing

The sides of the fingers, one of the most sensitive parts of the body, are often skipped over in massage. Awaken them with this stroke.

Using both of your hands, weave all of your fingers between the fingers of one of your partner's hands — you decide what fits where — and bend the whole hand straight back at the wrist. Fifteen fingers and three hands bending back together feels, somehow, just right. You'll be surprised how many people have always wanted to try this.

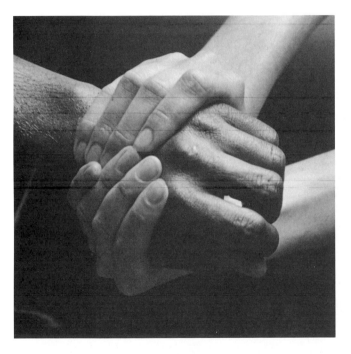
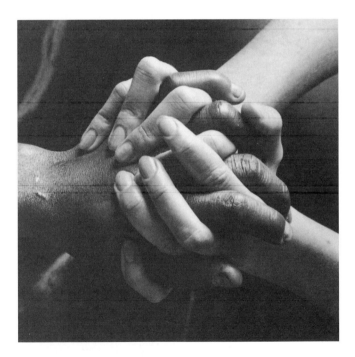

Pulling the Fingers

Just as you supported the arm in order to massage the hand, you must first support the hand to massage the fingers. Use a small pillow, or, while kneeling next to your partner's hand, fold his palm and fingers over your knee. Massage the fingers one at a time. Starting with the pinky and advancing across to the thumb, weave each one of your partner's fingers through your fingers (as shown). Grasp your partner's finger at the base and pull up the sides in a corkscrew motion. At the top end of the finger, make sure to pull off the nerve-rich sides. Pressing above and below the fingernail causes blood to squeeze against the sides of the fingers, a slightly unpleasant effect.

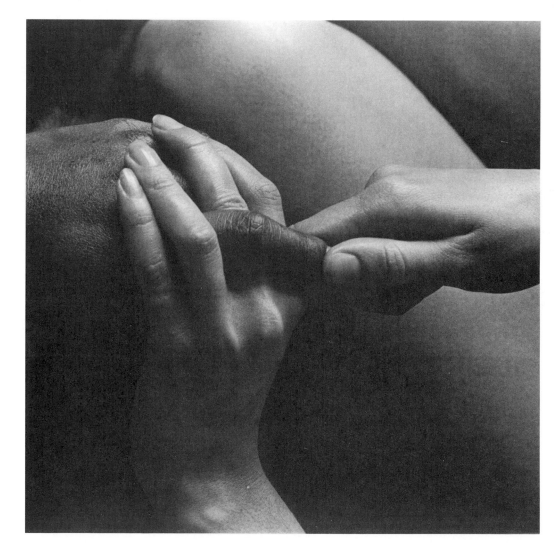

Thumb Kneading

Lifting your partner's hand to massage it will elevate part of the forearm. On a thin massage surface, you may want to provide extra arm support with a small pillow just below the elbow. Lift your partner's arm above and below the elbow and move it onto the pillow. Observe the etiquette of massage: You do all the work; she should do nothing at all.

Using both of your hands to begin thumb kneading the back of the hand, grip the palm side with four fingers. Your thumbs will then travel freely over the back of the hand, onto the carpal ligament at the wrist, and, finally, halfway up the forearm. Make sure the back of the wrist gets plenty of attention. Unlike on the opposite side of the hand, where surface blood vessels compromise the stroke, thumb kneading here reaches the full width of the ligament. Glide over the eight tiny bones just beneath the skin.

Use the whole surface of your thumbs whenever possible, moving to fingertip strokes only on the edges of the hand. Rotate your thumbs in broad circles, one thumb up while the other is down. Feel the smooth skin and bone ripple beneath your thumbs. The stroke advances in small deliberate steps all the way from the base of the fingers to the forearm. Spend extra time on the wrist going and coming, circling back and forth a dozen times or more over the carpal ligament with the tips of your thumbs.

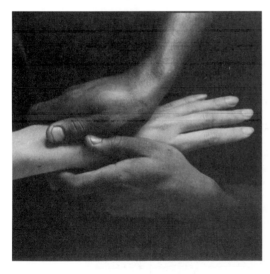
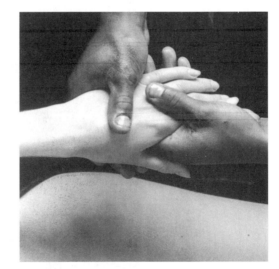

Hand-Over-Hand Stroking

This high intensity circulation movement, a variation of the fast stroking techniques you used on the legs, adds a dramatic flourish to your hand massage. Over the past few minutes, a small but significant fluid release effect has been set in motion across the fingers and palm. Use this stroke to clear acidic irritants from the hands and refresh your partner. It spreads warmth from the fingertips to the wrist.

Start on the back of your partner's hand (as shown). Bend your fingers to fit around the sides of her hand and be ready to form them to the shape of her forearm as you move up off the hand. Press forward across the wrist in short hand-over-hand strokes with one hand following close behind the other. Lead with your pinky, pressing down at a slight angle. The front hand lifts the moment the back hand makes contact. Bring the pinky of your contact hand down right behind the thumb of the front hand. Maintaining the same brisk hand-over-hand motion, continue moving forward halfway up the forearm.

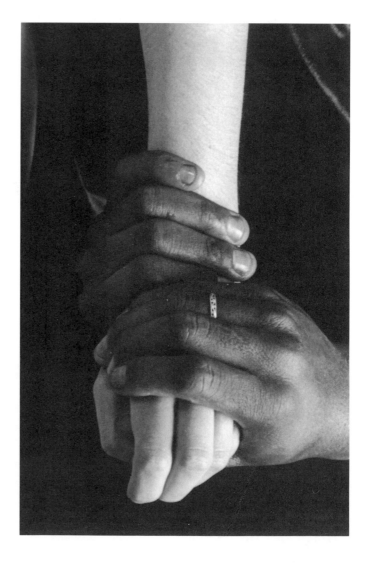

Pulling Off the Hand

End your hand massage with a two-part sequence that creates a waterfall of sensation from the forearm to the fingertips. Here again, be generous; it makes the hands feel important.

Start on the middle of the forearm, holding the arm between your thumb and fingers. As you begin to pull down to the fingertips with one hand, bring the other hand up to grasp the middle forearm. The hands descend one after another, pulling across the forearm, wrist, hand, and finally the fingers. At the end, this full-hand stroke turns into a fingertip movement. Break contact with your partner's fingertips at the same moment you make contact on the forearm with the other hand.

Brushing the Hands

Your final stroke on the hands, a light hand-over-hand brushing from the forearm to the fingertips, lets your partner experience waves of exquisitely light sensation over the whole area you've just massaged. Brush down the arm in an unhurried series of hand-over-hand strokes, some long, covering the whole distance from the forearm to the fingertips, and others that concentrate on a single spot. Both long and short brushing strokes should descend slowly from the forearm to the fingers. Finally, pull off the hand until only your fingertips are touching your partner's fingertips. Hold that contact for a silent count of ten, then, just as you break contact the final time, reach up with your free hand and take hold of the shoulder. Move the feeling from the hands to a spot just below the head.

Maintaining even contact with the shoulder, move to a comfortable spot above your partner's head where you will begin the final part of the full-body massage.

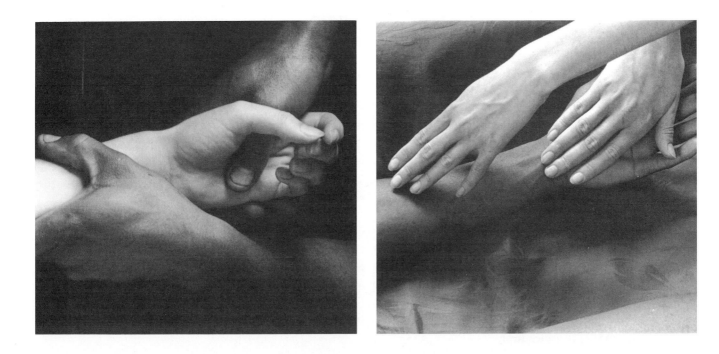

CHAPTER II

The Head & Face

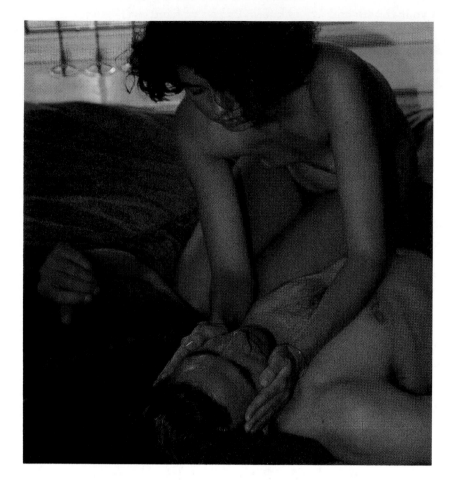

You start to see your partner differently during massage. As you begin head massage, look closely at the size relationship among your partner's head, neck, and shoulders. Think of the head as a large, heavy object that must be supported by the neck and shoulder muscles throughout the day. If she has tiny shoulders and does sedentary work requiring that the head be held in position for hours at a time, she probably experiences neck and shoulder pain, even headaches, throughout the day. The strokes that follow will soothe the head by relaxing the supporting muscles first.

Every other part of the body requires that you move from one side of the body to another to massage it properly. The entire head, however, can be massaged from directly above (including, with minor changes, the facial strokes that are shown here done from below).

Neck and shoulder tension are transmitted directly to the fine muscles of the face, particularly the highly flexible tiny muscles of expression. We all know how quickly tension becomes visible on the face; however, it can disappear as fast as it appears.

The second part of head massage is the massage facial, a four-minute beauty treatment that can actually change the way your partner looks. Wrinkles, for example, have little to do with moisture content of the skin (which is why many of the expensive "antiwrinkle" creams are so disappointing). Fatigue of the subcutaneous muscles causes a visible collapse of the tissue on the surface of the face. Fortunately, those muscles respond quickly to massage. Try the strokes that follow and see for yourself.

Effective facial massage requires relaxed hands and feet. Tension virtually anywhere on the body will find its way to the muscles of expression. If your partner suffers from tight muscles running parallel to the spine, for instance, the whole back will be tense. Large upper back muscles, that support the head will then tug on facial muscles, which are tuned to register the most subtle nuances of feeling. You won't see your partner's face become peaceful until the rest of the body is relaxed.

Most of the effects of good massage are internal and personal. But for the muscles of expression on the face, the dramatic changes that take place during massage could remain entirely secret. A relaxed face is the badge of a good full-body massage.

HEADACHE

♦ The next time your partner turns up with a headache or stiff neck, give head massage a chance before you reach for the pain pills.

Unlike the rest of the body, the head can be massaged from a standing or sitting position while your partner lies on a bed with her head near the edge. Do everything you can to make her whole body comfortable before you start. Pillows under the knees will relax her abdominal muscles.

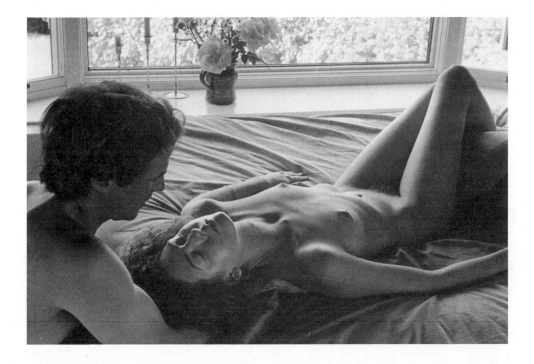

♦ Head massage always feels better if you start by vibrating under the shoulder blades.

Focus the first part of your head massage on the network of tissue surrounding the shoulder joint.

Vibrating the Chest and Shoulders

Give the shoulders plenty of attention before massaging the head. We have seen how the head is supported by powerful muscles that originate in the upper back. No part of the body is more dependent on the condition of nearby tissues. Whether you want to banish a headache, combat facial wrinkles, or eliminate a stiff neck, head massage must begin around the shoulders. Start by gently vibrating the nerves that supply the head at their point of origin under the shoulder blades.

With your partner's head and shoulders well supported — by pillows, if necessary — get comfortable at a point directly above the head. Slide your hands straight under the muscular top of the back, keeping your fingers extended straight ahead. Let his head fall back between your arms. At the shoulder blades, bend your fingers straight up. Keeping them rigid, push up and down about twice a second against your partner's back. Pull back slowly as far as the shoulder tops while you vibrate. Don't try to reverse the stroke at the shoulders, simply reposition your hands and begin pulling back once again. Three to six repetitions of this simple stroke help the muscles above to relax during head massage.

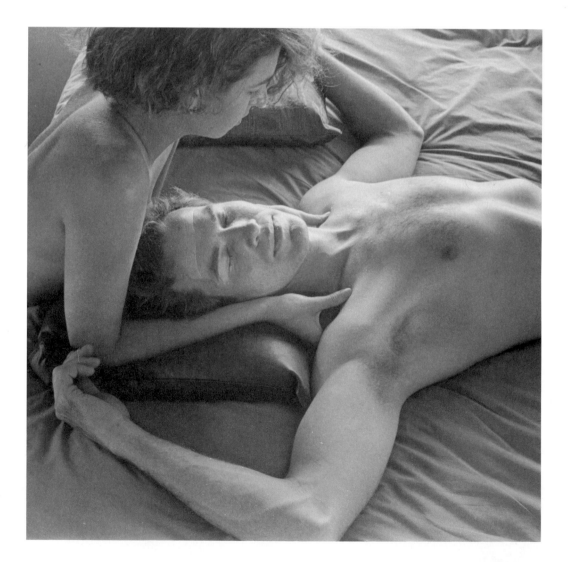

Circling the Neck

Neck massage focuses on the muscles along the spine, without pressing down on the spine itself. Circling directly on the muscles of the neck delivers what television drug ads promise: instant relief for all kinds of nasty aches and pains. People with stiff necks can't get enough of it.

Reach in under your partner's neck with four fingers of each hand held tightly together. Point your fingertips at each other and let the spine fill the gap between them. Now, rotate your hands in small ascending circles, pressing up against the neck as you turn. Start just above the shoulders and move up slowly toward the base of the skull. At the center of the base of the skull you will find a soft depression, just big enough to admit two or three fingers of each hand. Turn your hands until the fingers are extended straight forward and bent slightly (as shown). This is the spot where the spine and every one of the thirty-one pairs of nerves that supply the body emerge from the brain. The brain itself feels nothing; sensation begins right under your fingertips. Gently press inward while you circle up and down with each hand. Your little fingers will brush each other just below the skull.

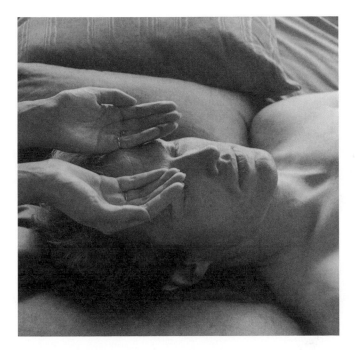
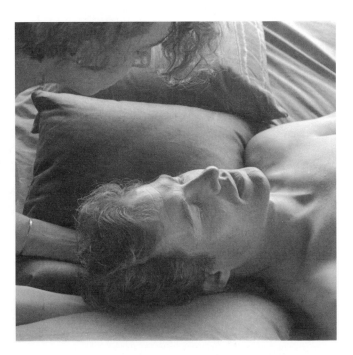

Flexing the Neck

Flex the neck from above. Surely the human head didn't evolve into its current shape in order to make massage more convenient, but it's tempting to imagine such a scenario after trying this stroke. The head has two natural handles that make turning and rotating it nearly effortless. Reach around to the back of the head and grasp the marked indentation at the base of the skull. Wrap your other hand around your partner's chin. Hold both "handles" firmly and simply pull straight backward, exerting equal pressure on the back of the skull and the chin. Your partner's head will move smoothly from side to side as you turn your hands. Watch to be sure the chin remains level as you turn; if it doesn't, you're pulling harder with one hand than the other.

First, test the limits of this passive exercise and train your partner's head to accept them. Carefully, turn the head to one side until you feel resistance, then turn to the other side. Remember where you encountered the points of tension on both sides. Rotate the head in a level arc from one point of tension to the other, pulling straight back as you turn. Do three complete back-and-forth neck flexing cycles, then gradually release your chin and skull grips. Let your partner feel the difference between neck massage and everything else.

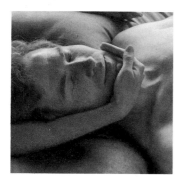

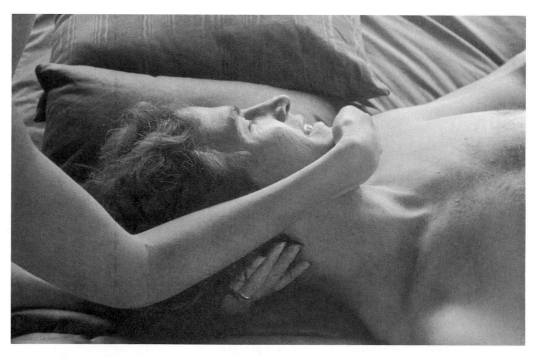

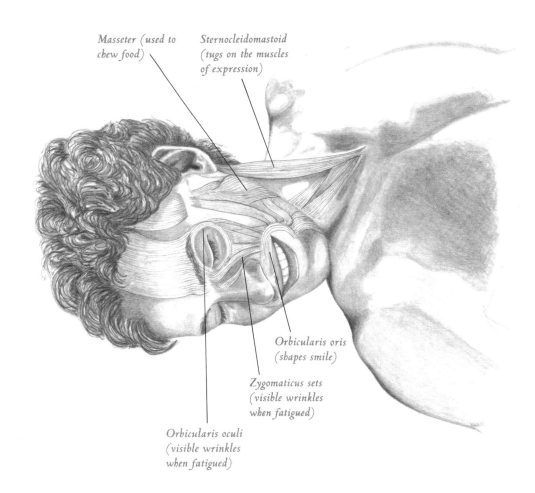

Masseter (used to chew food)

Sternocleidomastoid (tugs on the muscles of expression)

Orbicularis oris (shapes smile)

Zygomaticus sets (visible wrinkles when fatigued)

Orbicularis oculi (visible wrinkles when fatigued)

The vertebrae of the neck, unlike those below, have little lateral support. Crushed together, at the mercy of gravity all day long, they must bear the full weight of the head without help. Nerves supplying every part of the body pass through these vertebrae. Direct pressure on the nerves causes muscle spasm and a spreading soreness across the shoulders and upper back.

The results are transmitted directly to the surface of the face. Large neck muscles pulling hard from below distort the delicate muscles of expression.

Neck flexing reverses the forces on the neck, opening up the vertebrae and stretching cramped muscles. First, your partner smiles, then you see the difference on his face.

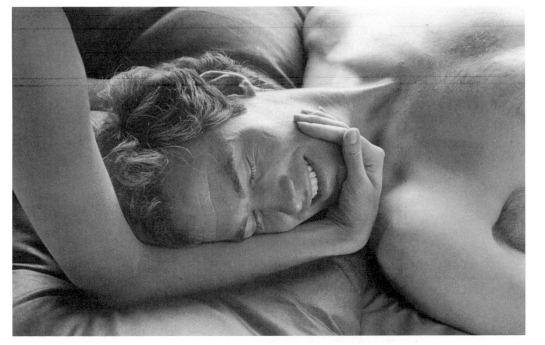

Tension Test

This simple test tells you how your face massage is going — without interrupting the massage to ask. Press straight down on the chin. If your partner's mouth opens easily, he's relaxed. If you feel resistance, don't force the jaw or call his attention to the fact. Repeat your kneading and friction sequences, focusing on the back of the jaw, then try the test again. More massage will bring peace to the face.

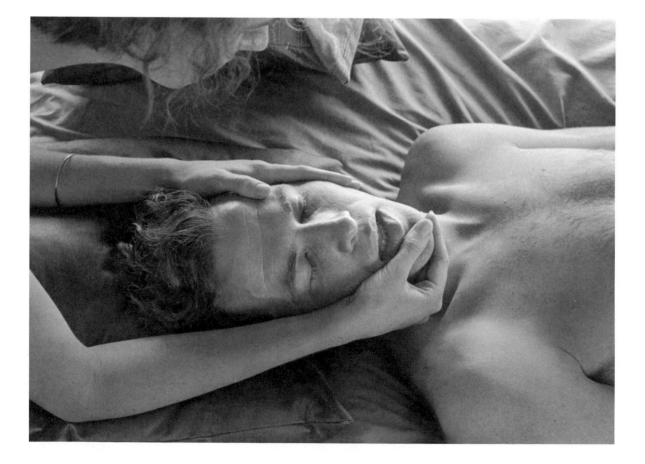

Scalp Friction

Massage the scalp before you massage the face. Tightness at the top of the head will pull on muscles below, creating a kind of subliminal tension across the face. You'll see a visible difference in your partner's expression after a good scalp vibration.

Reach through your partner's hair with all ten fingertips firmly against the scalp. The fingers should remain in place while the scalp moves. Don't rub against the surface of the scalp. Press down until you feel the skin shifting back and forth over the skull. Reposition your fingers every half minute or so until you have spread vibration to every part of the scalp. Tight scalp muscles surrender tension quickly — you'll feel a greater range of movement in minutes.

SHINY HAIR

♦ This stroke also stimulates the subcutaneous blood vessels of the scalp, which supply the roots of the hair. Oxygenating the scalp gives the hair a vibrant, glossy look.

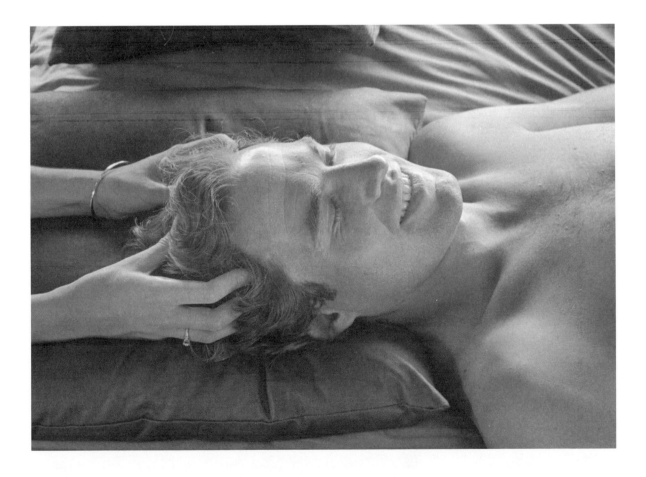

Circling the Temples

On the side of the face, just below the corners of the eyes, you will feel a bony circle with a depression at the center, directly over the temples. Feel for the temples with your fingertips, then massage them — first, one at a time, then both at once.

Usually three or four fingers will fit against the temples. Anchor the stroke on one side of the face (as shown) and feel for the opposite temple with your fingertips. Rotate about once per second inside the circle of bone. Then, press against the temples on both sides of the face and rotate your fingers in symmetrical circles three times in each direction. Vary the stroke by turning your fingertips in opposite directions. Keep the circles light and rhythmic. Press down on the center of the forehead with your thumbs during the last few revolutions.

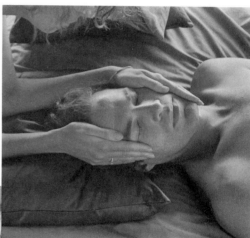

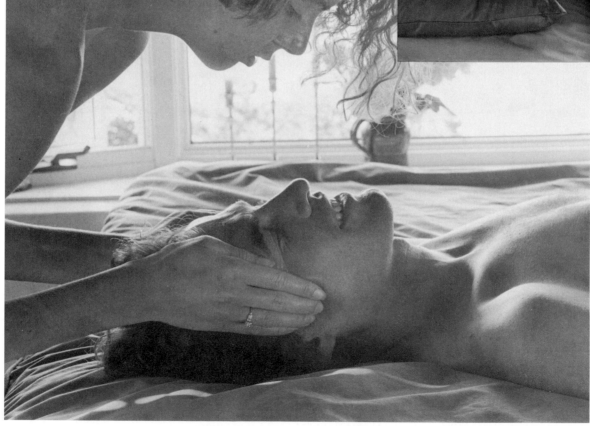

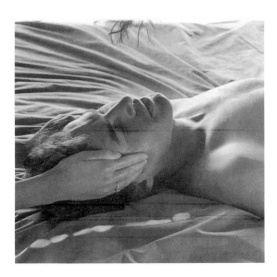

Unlike every other part of the body, the face is linked, via direct nerve paths, to the brain. You don't need deep strokes to make an impression. The face is an exquisitely sensitive area — your lightest touch will be noted.

Sensation zones on the chest, legs, hands, and feet connect to spinal vertebrae on the back, then to the brain. Facial sensation zones, more an extension of the brain itself, make the head a perfect place to end a full-body massage. Every touch seems magnified here. Temple strokes make contact at the center of the face's three sensation zones.

All these branches of the facial nerve merge at the center of the skull, where they connect directly to the brain.

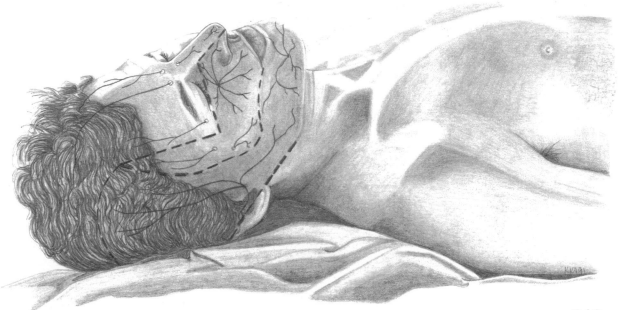

♦ Strokes on the shoulder and neck drew your partner's attention to the intimate tactile connection among the head, shoulders, and back. You needn't say a word; your hands make the point.

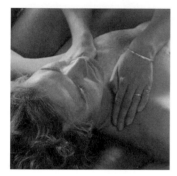

Stroking the Face

While stroking the face, extend sensation from the forehead to the chest, another natural connection. Take your time. During this stroke, your partner experiences one of the most tender moments in massage.

Press the full flat surface of both hands against the sides of your partner's face, allowing your fingertips to rest against the temples. The temples become a cen-

tral point for massage of the face. Pull down slowly across the cheeks and let your fingers mold themselves to the shape of his jaw. Use very light pressure on the sides of the neck above the surface blood vessels. Continue pulling straight down onto the top of the chest. Stop there with your thumbs touching (as shown). Hold the midchest contact for a silent count of ten, then start down again from the forehead.

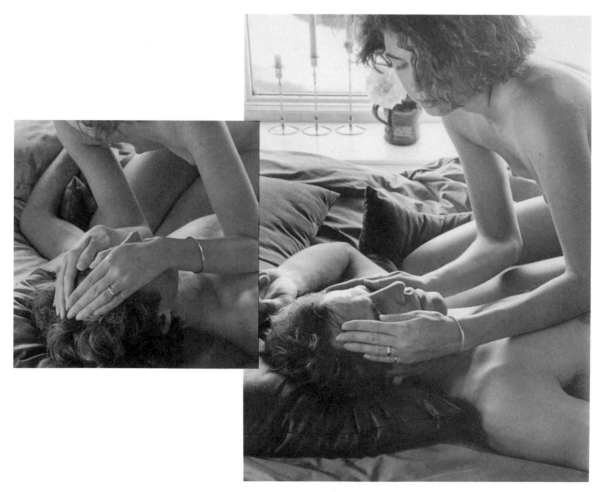

Stroking the Forehead

The first of several intense forehead movements, stroking creates a downward wavelike sensation on the top of the face. It stimulates circulation in the sinuses, which leaves the head feeling light and clear.

Cup your hand to fit across the forehead from temple to temple. Starting just below the hairline, use a hand-over-hand motion to stroke straight down across the forehead. Change to superficial pressure on the bridge of the nose. As one hand lifts off the bridge of the nose, the other presses down at the top of the forehead. One hand is up while the other is down — never break contact with the face.

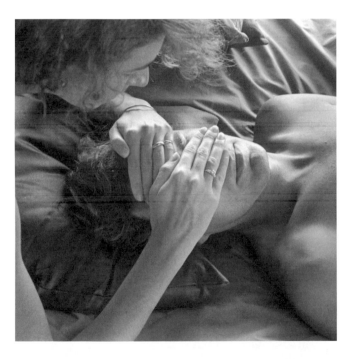
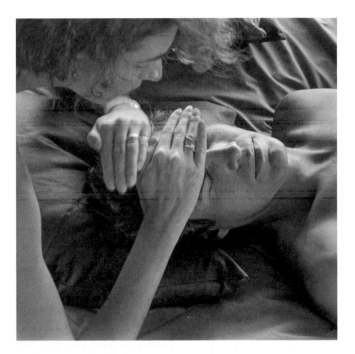

Pressing the Forehead

Forehead massage takes place on the body's only bare skin located directly over the brain. Perhaps that explains its peculiar intensity. No stroke in massage commands more attention. For once, you are no longer at the mercy of remotely controlled muscles or tortuous nerve paths. Here, nothing but a thin layer of skin and bone stands between your partner's brain and the intoxicating feeling.

Curve your hands to fit the precise contour of your partner's forehead. Your fingertips rest near one temple, while the heel of your hand contacts the opposite one. Press down evenly, using moderately strong pressure, across the whole surface of your hands. Hold your maximum pres-

sure position for a silent count of thirty, then release it slowly.

At first, the strongest feeling spreads across the center of your partner's forehead, midway between the hairline and the eyes. To focus pressure near the temples, rest your elbows on the massage surface and press in from the sides (as shown).

Press down three times each on the front and sides of the forehead, taking care to release pressure gradually each time. The whole face seems to surrender its tension each time you apply pressure. You will return to this stroke again and again during facial massage.

Pain turns to pleasure under your hands. Listen as you press down. Soft delighted moaning means the headache has vanished.

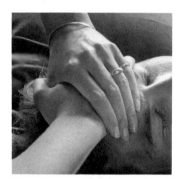

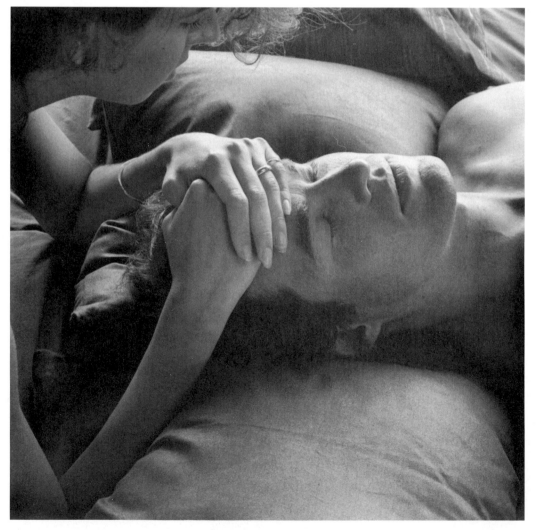

Forehead Compression

This compression stroke, a variation of forehead pressing, directs pressure to a single spot at the center of the forehead, usually, just what your partner wants after a few minutes of more general forehead pressing.

Lace your fingers together (as shown) and press straight down with both hands a few inches above the top of the nose. Circle slowly, on the surface of the forehead, first in one direction, then the other.

♦ The face has a way of surrendering its tension all at once. Watch for this dramatic change during forehead compression. If you don't see it, use this stroke to build an extended facial massage focused on your partner's muscles of expression. Add forehead stroking, scalp friction, and frequent temple stroking to the strokes on the next two pages. Return to forehead compression every minute or two. With so little area to cover, it's easy to mix and blend strokes on the face. Let the movements flow into each other so your partner never feels an abrupt starting and stopping. Massage the jaw again if the tension test is difficult. Stroke the face, flex the neck, vibrate the shoulders and keep pressing the forehead.

Tension is an unnatural state. Give your partner's face some time to relax during your facial massage, and it will.

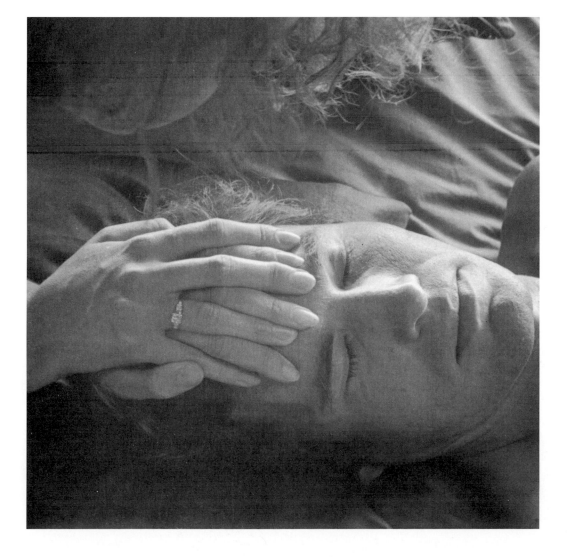

◆ Tension freezes the face; massage animates it. This rotating stroke shows your partner just how plastic the face can be, and how massage works to unlock facial muscles.

Rotating the Cheeks

While pressing against the sides of the face with the full surface of your palms and fingers, rotate your hands in slow opposing circles. After three revolutions, reverse the circles. As your partner's cheeks roll to follow your fingers, you will see a rubbery distorted expression followed, usually, by a broad smile.

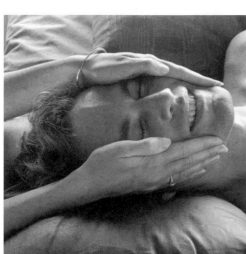

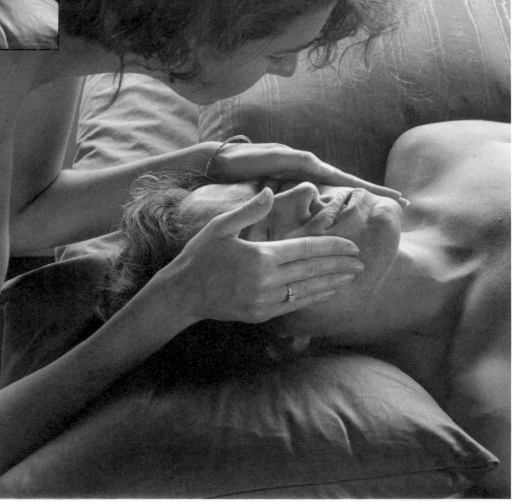

Jaw Friction

When the powerful jaw muscles become tense, the rest of the face is sure to follow. If your partner's mouth doesn't open easily, try this fingertip friction variation on the muscles that keep it clamped shut. This fingertip friction stroke supplies direct pressure to tensed jaw muscles on both sides of the face.

Apply friction on one side of the face while anchoring the head with the full surface of your other hand (as shown). Press down lightly with the thumb of your anchor hand on the center of your partner's forehead. With your friction hand, feel carefully for the outline of your partner's mouth; note the muscular ridge at the back. Start rotating your fingers in small circles just below the corner of the mouth and work back to the muscular ridge, roughly, below the corner of the eye. Here, at the thickest part of the jaw muscle, tension creates visible knotting. Press down firmly while you turn. Direct fingertip friction will relax the jaw and, with it, the face itself.

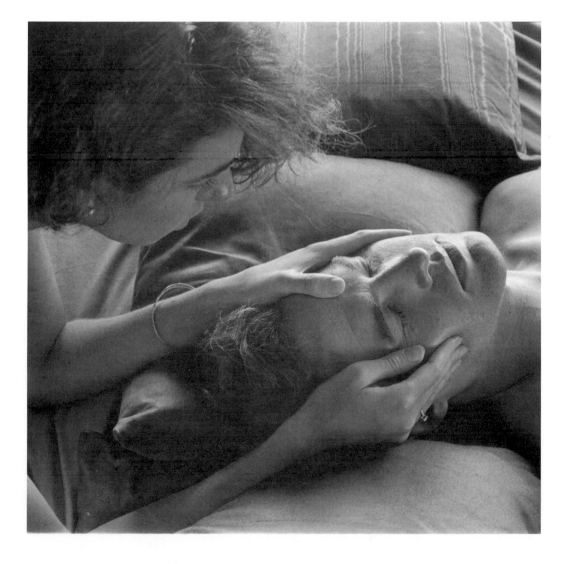

THE FINISHING TOUCH

♦ Breaking contact with the final fingertip concludes your full-body massage — take your time.

Ending A Massage

End your full-body massage on the forehead, directly over the brain. First, make contact with both hands on the center of the forehead as though you were about to repeat the compression movement. This time, however, turn your hands until the fingertips cross and press straight down moderately hard without moving your hands from side to side. Hold your maximum pressure for a silent count of thirty. Then, slowly lift your hands until only your fingertips are touching the skin. Break contact at the fingertips one by one leaving just a single fingertip (you choose the one) touching your partner's forehead. After experiencing tactile luxuries everywhere on the body, your partner's attention finally narrows to a single point at the center of his forehead.

Press down for a silent count of ten, then lift your fingertip straight up and away from your partner's body. The full-body massage is now complete. Leave the massage area quietly and let your partner decide when to move from the world of pure sensual pleasure to the other world we all know so well.

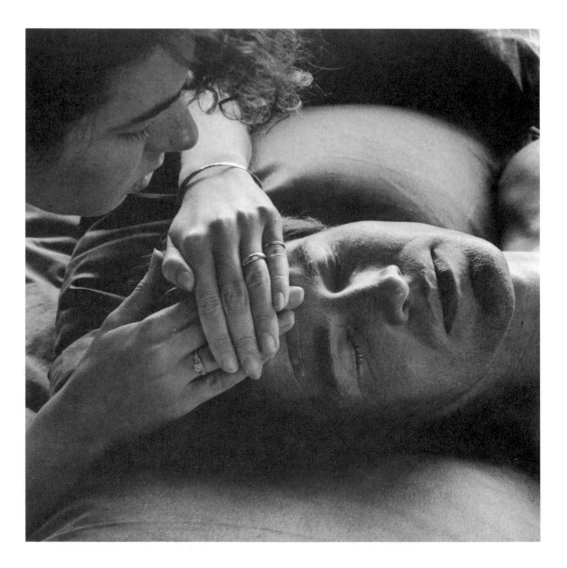

PART 3

Massage Specialties

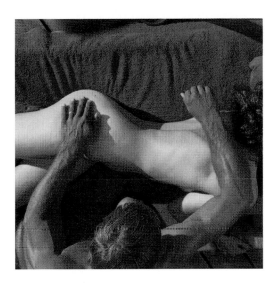

CHAPTER 12

Erotic Massage

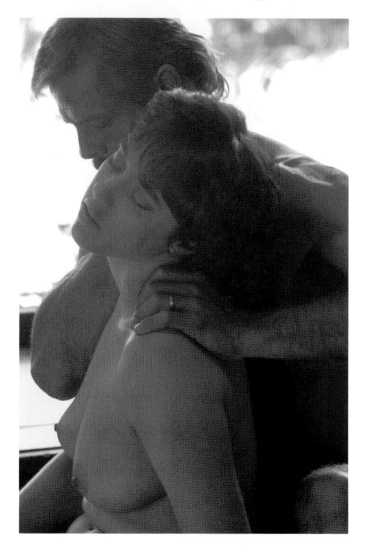

This chapter does not provide a course in seduction techniques or an arsenal of sexual ammunition for the rejected lover. How uncomplicated life would be, if massage could always ignite the fires of uncontrollable lust in the object of your desire. Alas, the feelings must be mutual. Before you begin, ask yourself: Am I about to massage a partner or a lover? Since attraction always precedes sexual desire, you really shouldn't expect to make love to somebody who doesn't care for you.

However, once the attraction is apparent, combining massage with sex magnifies the power of both experiences. If you have been searching for an aphrodisiac, a way to ignite your sex life, try this.

Don't confuse erotic massage with foreplay. The door to the sensual world will remain closed until your lover is relaxed and ready. Yes, you can always fast forward into sex, but the experience may be disappointing. Massage will relax your partner's body first, and if you want to prolong the pleasure of sex, nothing else matters more. Erotic massage begins with basic techniques for eliminating stress, perhaps the major obstacle to good sex. Relaxation may take some time but every minute you will be giving pleasure with your hands. Let your lover direct the first part of your erotic massage, focusing strokes on aches and pains in the back and shoulders and tight muscles throughout the body. For now, simply let sensual massage become a stronger reality than stress.

Once you've relaxed your lover, sensual massage turns erotic, intensifying pleasure for both of you and creating a sultry mood that lasts for hours. First, you broaden the range of sensation, then you amplify individual sensations. By awakening sensually deprived parts of the body, you give your lover "permission" to feel from head to toe. She starts living in her body, feeling things deeply, not only with the so-called erogenous zones — maybe 5% of the body — but with the whole body. Your toes have a right to an erotic experience; so does your scalp.

Erotic massage is one of life's great pleasures — you owe it to your lover (and yourself) to create the experience. Your goal is simple: to bring your partner to a point, before sex, where she thinks: "This is the most wonderful thing I've ever felt — what else is there in life?"

Then she finds out.

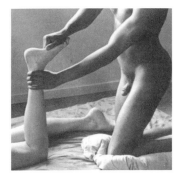
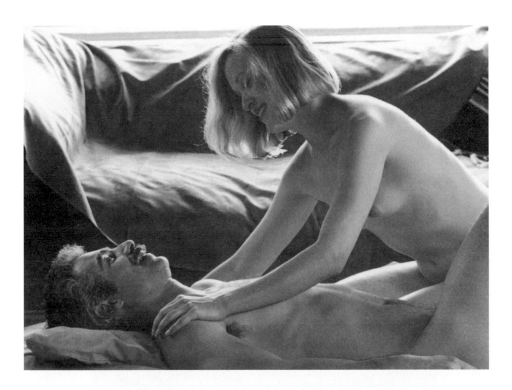

♦ Forget most of what you've learned about how to behave in bed.

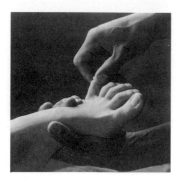

Basic Fireworks

Erotic massage turns sex into a sensual feast, which is only fair: If you're not generous with your partner during sex, when will you be? Prepare for the feast by firmly rejecting the fast food approach: routinely rubbing your partner's body a few inches away from the genitals while methodically working toward orgasm.

Instead, move sensation out to the sensually starved parts of the body; for now, the genitals will take care of themselves. You will give up nothing during erotic massage, you will only add to the possibilities.

Let's play. Forget most of what you've learned about how to behave in bed . . . or during massage. You can now talk while you massage, eat, drink, smoke, whistle, or dance. You can dress up like Louis XV and order oysters to be flown in from a nearby city. You can stand on the furniture and play with dolls. In other words, there are no rules. If you can't be free during sex, when will you be?

Make freedom your goal and use massage to get there. Say, your lover is afraid to feel unusual sensations . . . or any sensations on certain parts of the body. Don't panic. We are taught to ration our pleasures, or deny them altogether. If your partner practices pleasure censorship, you can use massage to liberate her body. In fact, massage is becoming an important tool for therapists who seek to develop a patient's sexuality. Long-shut doors swing open; people change permanently.

Before beginning erotic massage, you may want to visualize a few possibilities. If trying something different frightens your lover, spend a few minutes dreaming together. Talk about your desires and imagine acting them out — let your subconscious become conscious. Think of erotic massage as play, even fantasy, instead of methodology. You have a combination that even the pampered rich cannot better: your educated touch and your lover's body. Dim the lights, turn on some quiet music, and place your oil nearby.

If ever mind and body will merge for your lover, they will do so now.

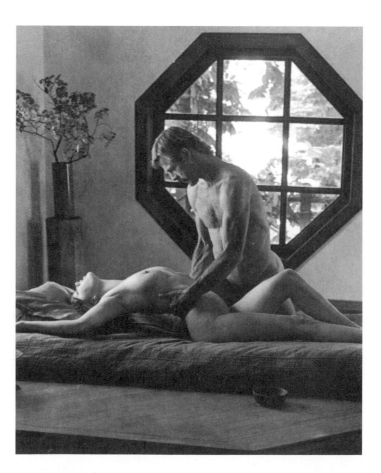

The Erotic Foot

Think of the feet as symbols of the abandoned body. Like the elbows, back of the knees, and hands, feet are generally ignored during lovemaking; they become casualties of hurried sex. Whose idea was it to *save time* during sex, as though your lover was a piece of candy, an object of instant gratification? The peculiar pleasure censorship practiced so widely in our puritanical society encourages us not to dwell on good feelings. If sex is about release, not extended pleasure, we can rush through the so-called "erogenous zones" and make contact with 5 or 10% percent of the body. Erotic massage takes a more satisfying approach: find out what your lover actually wants and give it to her.

The body's desire to be touched is a fundamental need, and denying it during sex can be almost as demoralizing as physical hunger. Erotic massage derives its wonderful power by combining a playful approach with scrupulous attention to detail. Use the techniques that follow to delight your lover's senses on every part of the body. Take your time during erotic massage — nothing else matters more — and let your lover savor each moment. Whole-body sex, sweet and luxurious. Start with the feet.

Foot massage allows you to prolong the pleasure of sex by setting an unhurried pace at the beginning. Fingertip kneading strokes travel effortlessly around the nooks and crannies of the foot. Reach into the depression of the arch and below the ankles with the tips of your thumbs. Turn the foot and knead both sides. Press the ball of your lover's foot against your knee (for support) and push up toward the heart with a firm hand-over-hand circulation stroke. Brush both feet at once with your fingertips. Move the feeling from her ankles to her toes, a few inches. So much feeling for such a short distance.

♦ Pleasure censorship denies your partner the luxury of experiencing his own feelings. Sex, eating, sports, even relaxation are habitually rushed, lest they be enjoyed too much.

Foot massage trains the body's most ignored muscles to relax and yield to pleasure. Unlike tension and pain, pleasure can be recalled long after it is experienced.

By allowing your partner to experience pleasure in unexpected places, foot massage animates the body.

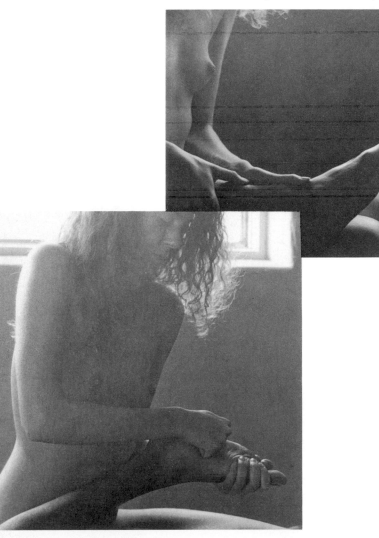

The Headache Solution

The most common impediment to good sex is tension. Attempting to ignore your lover's tension during a sexual encounter will probably make her irritable. And using sex itself to relax a tensed body relaxes the wrong partner. Never ignore your partner's feelings, especially when they are negative. With massage, you can turn a problem into an opportunity.

Don't surrender to common headaches. Whether or not your partner's headache is due to mental or physical causes, you can work through the body to get rid of it.

The general muscle tightening and impeded blood flow that accompanies stress devastates the head. During vasoconstriction, powerful muscles across the shoulders and the top of the back clamp down on the nerve and blood vessel bundle that supplies the head. The bloodless complexion of headache victims is a direct consequence of this pressure. This stroke breaks the vicious circle of stress with a single super lift that literally dumps blood directly into the brain.

Like the waist lift (see page 96), this stroke elevates your partner's body from the base of the spine. But this time you must go beyond merely flexing the lower back and lift high enough to bring your lover's whole body into the air (as shown). Needless to say, this stroke isn't for everyone, but it's not as difficult as it looks. First, use your outside leg as a tripod, lifting your knee and planting your foot next to your lover before you begin. Then, lift straight up until her head falls back. Hold at the top of the lift for a silent count of thirty or more. You can see the blood rushing into the head and oxygenating the brain. And your lover can feel it.

Follow the lift with concentrated kneading around the neck and shoulders to relax the muscles that support your partner's head. Circle on the temples and press the forehead — long, deep pressing. Bring your hands up slowly from your lover's forehead. She will follow you back into this world.

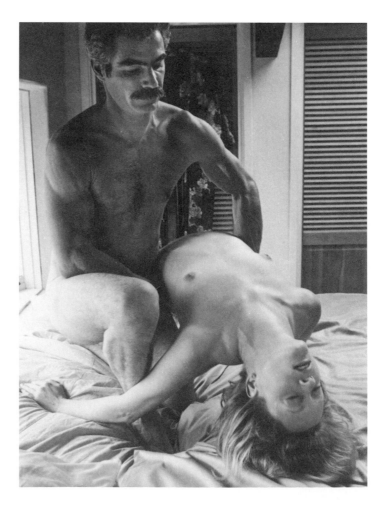

Twisting the Body

You can bet that your lover secretly enjoys being twisted into unusual shapes, especially if you do all the work. When she sits up, her shoulders become natural handles for flexing the upper body; handles that have probably never been used . . .

Sit directly behind her for this stroke. Make a fist while bending your right arm at the elbow. Pull back on the front of her right shoulder with your forearm, while pushing forward on her left shoulder with your left hand. Twist the shoulders to the point of tension, hold for a silent count of ten and release slowly. After three twists, reverse the stroke, pulling back on the left shoulder while pushing forward on the right.

With your partner lying on her side, you can twist the whole body. Bend your elbow across her shoulder and push forward on her hips (as shown) to the point of tension, not beyond. Now reverse the stroke, pressing forward on the back of her shoulder with one hand while pulling back on the front of her hips with the side of your elbow.

Again, moaning means she likes it very much. Twist more.

Pulling the Body

The body's natural handles provide unexpected opportunities during an erotic sequence. Flexing the arm allows your lover to isolate sensation in her joint, a pleasant feeling especially when the arm floats up into the air while it happens.

Grasp her arm at the wrist and shoulder. While holding the shoulder firmly, pull up on the wrist. Rotate the arm while it's in this extended position.

Move from this to other passive exercises on the legs, hands, and feet. Pick up your lover's head and turn it. Allowing you to manipulate her body while she does nothing at all acknowledges your mutual trust. Compared to the random poking and probing that passes for foreplay, your informed touch has created a new mood.

Blend this stroke with slow friction movements at the joints. Knead her shoulders and hips with your fingertips. Let the feeling go on.

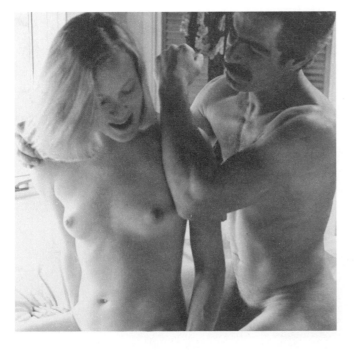
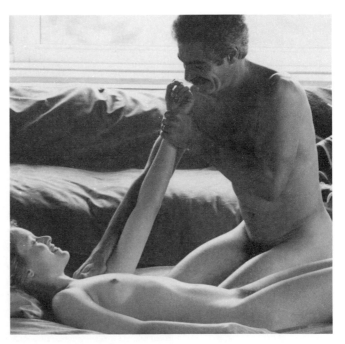

Side-Body Stroking

No matter what your instincts may tell you, the desire to be touched in unfamiliar places is stronger than ever during erotic massage. Side stroking proves that to your lover beyond a reasonable doubt.

Unlike on the front and back of the body, reclining on the side requires some small assistance from the muscles. For this reason, the sides of the body are generally massaged along the edges of the front and back during a full-body massage. Side-body massage is tacked on as an afterthought. Now you can place it center stage with a sweeping stroke that spreads deep sensation over a part of your partner's body that may have been ignored even during regular massage.

Oil the whole side, from shoulder to ankle, before you begin. Use extra oil to accommodate the various textures of the skin on the side of the body.

Start with your hands cupped over your partner's hip, thumbs touching. Move your hands away from each other at the same speed — one hand toward the shoulder, the other to the feet. Mold your fingers to the contour of your partner's side. Lean forward and reach up and down as far as you can. When you reach points near the shoulders and ankles, reverse the stroke and return to your starting position at the hips.

Your lover participates subtly in this movement by holding her body in position. This makes it easy for her to imagine the graceful sweep of this stroke while the two of you move together. Massage as dance.

Side-body stroking can easily be blended with the other full-body strokes. Ease your partner over onto her back or stomach and continue spreading sensation from one end of her body to the other.

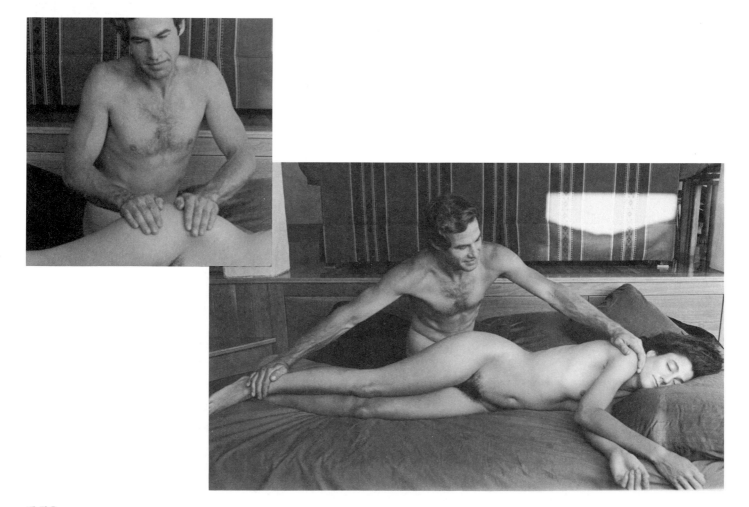

Oxygenating the Body

What a shame that the male chest, with its direct "window" to the lungs, receives so little attention during love-making. Moving back and forth across the top of the chest for just a few minutes with a variety of percussion movements will increase the oxygen content of the blood within the lungs by 10 to 15%. The lungs, in turn, recycle the whole blood supply of the body in less than a minute. Your partner will feel the effects of a super-oxygenated blood supply moments after you begin moving across the chest. Few strokes in massage have a more dramatic impact than percussion directly over the lungs.

This stroke sets up a gentle vibration that carries right through the chest, shaking loose debris in the lungs. Minutes after you begin, your partner will experience a spreading energized feeling. The area around the lungs seems warm and relaxed; not much later, the whole upper body begins to glow.

Make contact with your lover's chest with one hand (your contact hand) and use the other to apply percussion. Strike the back of your contact hand with the side of your closed fist about fifty times a minute. Move your contact hand around the chest as you strike it. Remember to break every "blow" at the wrist just before you reach the contact hand.

Move back and forth across your lover's chest for two or three minutes — more, if you're in the mood. Vary the stroke, if you like, with full-hand cupping (see page 49) or a light pinky snap (see page 49).

Your lover may be surprised at the unaccustomed contact; he may even laugh out loud, a sure sign he's enjoying himself. Keep up the percussion. He will probably ask you to continue when you stop.

Finish your lover's chest with a series of flat-hand circulation strokes over the whole area you've just stimulated. Oil the chest and side to the bottom of the rib cage. Add extra oil if his chest is hairy. Keeping your hands flat against his body, move down from the shoulders, across the chest, onto the side, and finally, back to the starting position. Ten of these easy-to-do circulation strokes will leave him feeling warm and relaxed.

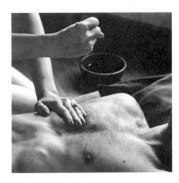

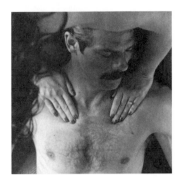

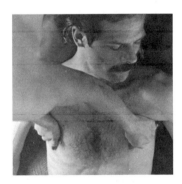

Clavicle bone

Sixth rib

Massage over the lungs up to the knobby, lower inside portion of the clavicle, and down to the sixth rib.

CHAPTER 13

Massage Toys and Resources

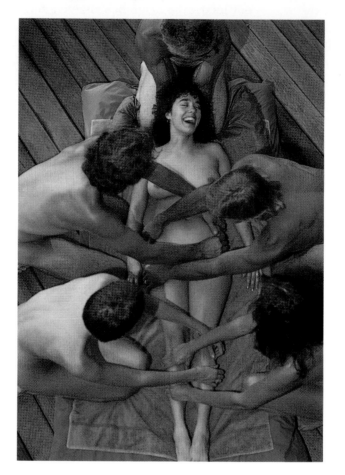

Don't read this section until you've fallen in love with massage. The basic requirements for good massage — a warm, quiet place and a few pennies' worth of vegetable oil — haven't changed for thousands of years. However, the recent massage explosion has given birth to a new group of merchants who understand, all too well, the American love of toys. With the right marketing, perhaps even massage can become a high-priced luxury requiring roomfuls of complex equipment. The Victorians invented steam-powered massage machines, which were meant to free people, once and for all, from the messy business of touching each other. The last twenty years have seen the reintroduction of self-massage chairs and automatic tables — souped up with servo motors and computerized "relaxation" programs. Throw a switch and you get jerked around relentlessly while hard knobby rollers are thrust against your body. You feel a sense of relief, if not relaxation, when it's over. For the most part, gadgetry just gets between your partner and the feeling, without providing a single memorable or enjoyable moment. Before you reach for your checkbook, think carefully about what you really need to do massage.

*F*irst, a few caveats. Pressing high-speed electrical devices against your partner's body will leave him (and your hand) numb. Massage oils that double as beauty treatments are usually nothing more than ordinary vegetable oil plus cosmetics, two substances that work better separately. At the high end of the massage toy spectrum, you can manage to spend hundreds of dollars on a racklike "massage chair," which promises to make possible a kind of instant massage in any setting. Take a course on how to use our chair, urges the manufacturer, then strap in a busy executive and start poking away at his body through layers of clothes. Attempts to rush, abbreviate, or somehow adapt the experience to the pressures of modern life change massage from a gourmet meal to a fast food.

Your own community probably has a professional masseur, a worthwhile profession if there ever was one, who stands ready to put a price on the experience itself. Don't hesitate to pay it if you have no other way to get a massage. After all, what good is money, if it doesn't make you feel good? But you shouldn't think of massage as a commodity that you must buy from others. Anyone who takes the time to learn, can do massage well; it's a minor skill, no more difficult than learning to use a knife and fork.

Once you've learned, you can play. These resources are meant to enhance the experience for the committed massage fan. The last one's free.

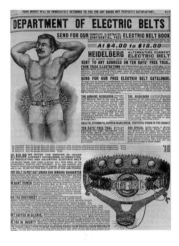

"Positively wonderful in its quick cure of all nervous and organic disorders arising from any cause, whether natural weakness, excesses, indiscretions, etc." — Sears, Roebuck catalogue, 1903.

Recommended: Somatron Lounge with six built-in body speakers driven by a full-range stereo. You recline on "floating resonator chambers." High density acoustic vibrations penetrate your body while you're massaged.

TouchAmerica, Inc., P.O. Box 1304, Hillsborough, N.C. 27278. Telephone: 1 (800) 678-6824.

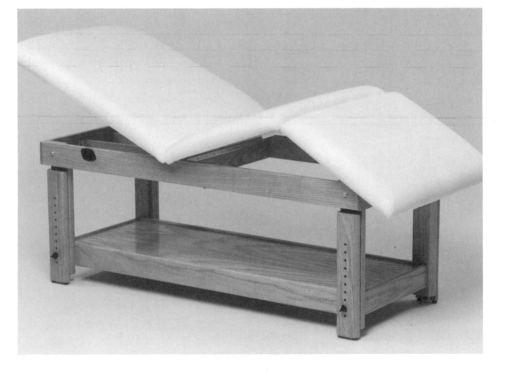

◆ Choose a professional masseur as carefully as you would a fine restaurant. Don't be afraid to make requests — it's your body. Feedback helps a masseur learn your preferences.

The Body Pad

Early on in massage you learn pillow tricks to accommodate male and female bodies. Setting up a comfortable massage surface and placing pillows wherever your partner's body needs extra support becomes a tricky part of your preparation and an ongoing concern for the next hour. Nevertheless, pillows have a way of missing the mark slightly or, worse, moving while you do massage. They also get bunched up, are easily lost, and don't travel well. Want to concentrate on massage instead of pillows?

Tim Owen, the masseur who designed the bodyCushion, a six-part system of adjustable soft supports, spent several years thinking about pillows, and it shows. His creation, a genuine pleasure to use, greatly simplifies doing massage on any surface. The system is guaranteed for five years and comes with a booklet of setup suggestions for various body types. It's neatly packed in a stylish knee-high tote bag, ready to go with you on the road.

The bodyCushion, Body Support Systems Inc., P.O. Box 337, Ashland, Oregon 97520. Telephone: I (800) 448-2400.

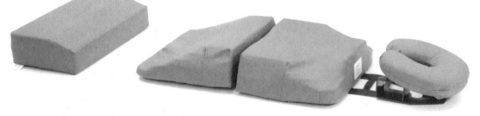

A Massage Table

We don't know whether the ancient Mediterranean civilizations developed an early bodyCushion, but we have located a few of their great stone massage tables, intact and ready to go after two thousand years underground — proving that the massage table, like the kitchen table, is one of the fundamental pieces of furniture in human life.

Basically unchanged for thousands of years, the massage table has now acquired folding legs in order to fit into taxis and airplane luggage compartments. A table simplifies your setup and allows you to do massage while standing, an easier position for long sessions. Adjustable legs bring your partner up to your waist, no matter what your height is. Living Earth Crafts makes exceptionally sturdy tables that are guaranteed for five years. They have easily adjustable legs as well as an adjustable face lift, an important feature that allows the table itself to take over support of the head at various angles. Use their table as is — or go one step further and put a bodyCushion on top.

Set up together, the two products will provide a nearly perfect massage surface virtually anywhere. Take them both on your next vacation and you will make friends everywhere you go.

Living Earth Crafts, 600 Todd Road, Santa Rosa, California 95407. Telephone: I (800) 585-2639.

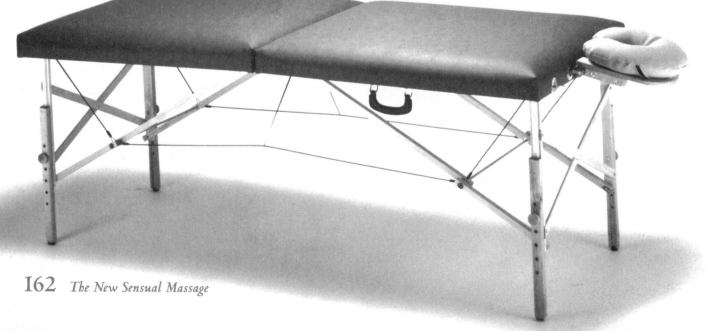

Massage Magazine

The voice of professional massage, every issue of *Massage Magazine* is packed with new techniques, as well as information on schools, licensing requirements, insurance, conventions, and trade organizations. Articles by masseurs from all over the world plus a contentious letters column help define this developing enterprise. Publisher-masseur Robert Calvert stretches the limits of massage with every issue.

NOAH Publishing Company, P.O. Box 1500, Davis, California. 95617-1500. Subscriptions: 1 (800) 533-4263.

Sensual Massage Video

Music, action, and massage. Watch a stroke, then try it for yourself. A classic massage, this video still feels as good as it did when it was screened at the Cannes Film Festival. See a whole-body massage unfold. Learn exactly what to do and when to do it. Six awards at international film festivals. In color; 50 minutes.

The Classic Art of Sensual Massage video.

Directed by Gordon Inkeles; cinematography by Bill Cote; original score by Michael Lobel.

Healing Arts Home Video, 312 Hampton Drive, Suite 203, Venice, California 90291. Telephone: 1 (800) 722-7347. In Canada, (416) 884-2323, BFS Ltd.

For information on Gordon Inkeles' lecture demonstration on massage, contact Schencke Associates, P.O. Box 220, Miranda, California 95553. Telephone: (707) 943-3600.

To relieve aching muscles during a triathlon, the world's largest massage team assembled on a perfect Hawaiian morning. You and I should have been there.

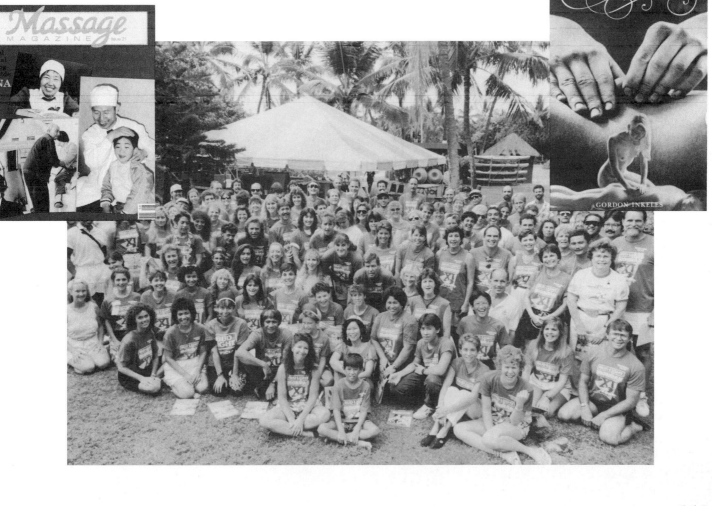

Group Massage

When massaging together, agree on the areas you want to cover before starting. Collisions and traffic jams, always a problem in crowded activities, can bring your group massage to a sudden, tangled halt. Begin a group session by deciding what part of the body each individual will massage.

By far, the most valuable resource in massage is other people. You've seen how much pleasure one pair of hands can provide — wait until you try four or five. Or nine. Nine pairs is close to the workable maximum for group massage, unless you are very big and can manage to find a group of very small people to massage you. The five pairs shown here turn out to be an ideal number for small parties.

You can cover your partner's body in much less time with a team, but why rush? This is your partner's introduction to one of life's great secret pleasures. Make it an evening of group massage.

Put an oil bottle near each masseur and keep a few towels handy. Scent the room with your partner's favorite essence. Music helps everyone concentrate on massage, instead of conversation.

In group situations, massage within a more limited range; no more than two feet in any direction. For opposite-side-of-the-body strokes, simply reach through each other's arms (as shown). The movements are identical to ordinary massage — but they all happen at once.

Agree on an informal plan before you start. You might decide to have two people massage both legs at once, while two others massage both arms. Everyone should start and end together with long circulation strokes, but the rest of group massage is up to you. Sometimes symmetry feels good. You might decide to knead together on both thighs, then do fingertip friction on the back of the knees. On the other hand, it's sometimes fun to vary your movements, stroking one side of the body while the other side is treated to mixed percussion. Both feet and both hands can be massaged at once while a fifth masseur works on the back. Or two people can knead the chest, while two others massage the head and feet, and a fifth kneads the legs. At a prearranged signal your partner can turn over and let the five of you massage the other side of her body.

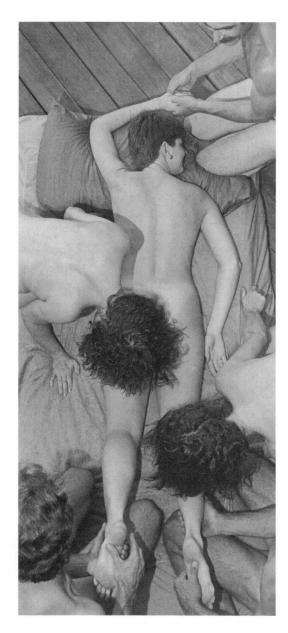

The Group Lift

Your partner hasn't been lifted into the air until she's been lifted by five or more friends at once.

Put the two strongest individuals at your partner's midsection. Lifting against the shoulder blades and hips, they will bear most of her weight. One person must support the head in a level position throughout the lift. The remaining two individuals lift above and below the knee (as shown). Everyone begins by sliding both hands under the body, palms up. Keep your fingers together and be silent. Be sure the group moves together.

Usually, five people will find it easy to lift one individual. Nevertheless, try lifting your partner just a few inches before you attempt the full-range stroke. If it seems difficult, bring in more lifters. Nobody should feel strained during this stroke.

Keep your palms flat and your fingers together. Bring your hands straight up, moving at a slow, even speed. Raise your hands in unison so your partner's body remains level. Lift her to a point slightly above your heads and lower your hands slowly to the starting position.

Lifts make unforgettable gifts, just right for your next special occasion. Your partner rises straight up into the air without the aid of a machine and without doing a single thing. She floats on a carpet of warm hands. Five people, ten hands, fifty fingers. In a single exuberant stroke, a group lift opens the door to the sensual world.

You know what to do to keep it open.

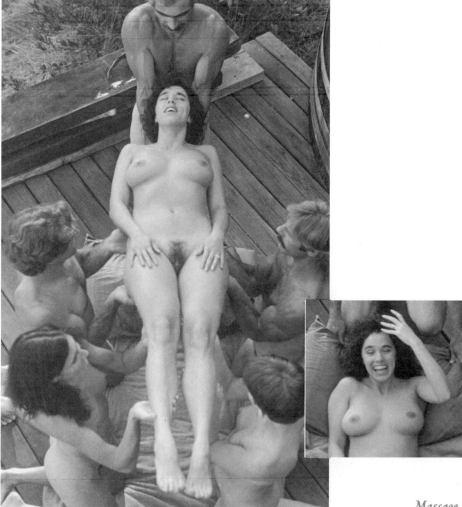